CLIENTS, CONSUMERS OR CITIZENS?

The Privatisation of Adult Social Care in England

Bob Hudson

First published in Great Britain in 2021 by

Policy Press, an imprint of
Bristol University Press
1–9 Old Park Hill
Bristol
BS2 8BB
UK
t: +44 (0)117 954 5940
e: bup-info@bristol.ac.uk

Details of international sales and distribution partners are available at
bristoluniversitypress.co.uk

British Library Cataloguing in Publication Data
A catalogue record for this book is available from the British Library

ISBN 978-1-4473-5569-4 hardcover
ISBN 978-1-4473-5570-0 paperback
ISBN 978-1-4473-5572-4 ePub
ISBN 978-1-4473-5571-7 ePdf

Cover design by Clifford Hayes
Front cover image: Freepik
Bristol University Press and Policy Press use environmentally responsible
print partners.
Printed and bound in Great Britain by CMP, Poole

Contents

Preface and acknowledgements   iv

Introduction   1

1   Before the market   7

2   The emergence and consolidation of the market   15

3   Dilemmas in the commissioning of adult social care   31

4   Dilemmas in the provision of adult social care   47

5   State or market?   63

6   Context: funding and administration   75

7   Looking ahead: an ethical future for adult social care   91

8   COVID-19: the stress test of adult social care   117

9   Conclusion: making it change – morals, markets and power   133

References   149

Index   179

Preface and acknowledgements

Writing this book has been both a personal and an academic journey. The Local Authority Social Services Act 1970 created new powerful local authority social services committees to plan, develop and deliver what we now call 'social care' for children and adults. In 1972 I was elected as a young councillor in Sunderland and served on the newly created committee. At the time it was assumed what was termed 'the personal social services' would follow the path to 'welfare state' status that had already been taken for health, education, housing and social security. There was much to commend this short-lived era though it was not without its faults and critics.

Today even the term 'social services' has vanished and the policy landscape has changed beyond recognition. Local authorities no longer make long-term plans, neither do they deliver services and support – that is largely the province of private companies. In the process there has been a complex shift in the way that we think about those requiring support to live their lives – a mix of client, consumer and citizen. Whereas fifty years ago I was a member of a working group developing a ten-yearear plan for local authority service expansion, today I am hunting around 'the market' trying to find a suitable and affordable care home for a family member. Politics, policy and the personal eventually intersect for all of us.

The book is not a diatribe about one approach or another, neither does it identify any simple solution; rather it seeks to untangle a complex story, to identify shifts and strands, continuities and discontinuities, problems and options. Putting it together has been hugely helped by so many excellent staff at Policy Press; from the first pitching of the idea right through to the final proofs, the team has worked like a well-oiled machine. My thanks to you all. Thanks also to those organisations and authors who have kindly given me permission to directly quote their work, and to the many scholars and practitioners whose work I have admired, utilised and referenced. And finally, a massive thank you my wonderful wife Val who has encouraged me to write this book. The contents are her life track too, from her time as a social worker in the 1970s and 1980s, a local authority social care manager in the 1990s and a social work academic afterwards.

The story is far from finished; indeed, it changes unceasingly. The initial framework on the balance between state, market and civil society was fundamentally changed by the advent of COVID-19. One of the consequences of the pandemic has been to thrust adult social care into the world of political tumult; change has been pledged but with no certainty of what it will be or where it will lead. Hopefully this book will help to make a modest contribution to the next stage of the policy journey.

Bob Hudson
May 2020

Introduction

This book is about 'adult social care' in England – the term commonly used to refer to personal care and practical support for older people and adults with physical disabilities, learning disabilities or mental health issues, as well as support for those caring for them informally. Much of the debate about adult social care tends to concentrate on the situation of older people, even though social care expenditure on adults of working age and older people is roughly equal in size. The focus is also on England. Although all parts of the UK have followed the same policy trajectory to some extent, this has become less so in the wake of devolution. While reference will be made to variations across the UK, this is not a comparative policy analysis. The terms 'personal care' and 'practical support' are also significant: the former is narrower than the latter, and both are restrictive compared to a wider concept such as 'well-being'. All of these definitions and their implications will be explored.

It is also a sector of considerable economic significance, enormous policy complexity and seeming political impenetrability. In terms of size, one recent estimate (IFC Consulting, 2018) put the total economic value of the sector at almost £50 billion. The workforce is estimated to be around 1.5 million – a massive source of employment. Moreover, it is estimated that if the adult social care workforce grows proportionally to the projected number of people aged 65 and over in the population, then the number of adult social care jobs will increase to around 2.2 million jobs by 2035 (Skills for Care, 2019). Better healthcare has also improved the life expectancy of people with physical and learning disabilities, meaning that more working-age adults are now in need of social care support. These adults are also less likely than older adults to have financial assets that disqualify them from receiving publicly funded care (NHS Digital, 2019b).

Political and policy responses to a sector of such significance have been contradictory. On the one hand, it has been subjected to massive ideological change in the way support is commissioned and delivered; on the other hand, the long-running debate around funding long-term care has been inconclusive. Since 1997, there have been more than a

1

dozen inquiries and government reports setting out a variety of ideas for funding social care in the longer term (House of Commons Library, 2019b). These include:

- 1999 – The government-appointed Royal Commission published its proposals, including a more generous means test and free personal and nursing care.
- 2009 – Labour's Green Paper proposed a National Care Service; a subsequent White Paper proposed the introduction of a two-year cap on social care charges initially, followed by free social care after 2015.
- 2011 – The Commission on the Funding of Care and Support set up by the Coalition government proposed a cap on lifetime social care charges and a more generous means test.
- 2014 – The Coalition government legislated to implement the commission's recommendations; however, in July 2015, the newly elected Conservative government postponed the introduction until 2016 and then postponed it indefinitely in 2017.

None of these proposals came to fruition, demonstrating the complexity of the problem and the extent to which it has become politically toxic. When the Labour Party proposed a new 10 per cent estate levy on death to fund their National Care Service proposals in 2010, this was described as a 'death tax' by the Conservative Party and was dropped during the campaign. Similarly, when the Conservative Party attempted to address the problem of 'catastrophic care costs' in the 2017 election campaign, this was dubbed 'a dementia tax' by the Labour Party and proved to be deeply unpopular.

In response, the 2017 Conservative government under Theresa May said that it would publish an adult social care Green Paper for consultation, and that this would cover not only how people paid for social care, but also a raft of other key issues. This seemed to be a welcome attempt to look at adult social care in the round rather than confining the debate to long-term funding. The then Secretary of State for Health and Social Care, Jeremy Hunt, went on to identify seven principles that would underpin this Green Paper:

- quality and safety embedded in service provision;
- whole-person, integrated care with the National health Service (NHS) and social care systems operating as one;
- the highest possible control given to those receiving support;
- a valued workforce;

- better practical support for families and carers;
- a sustainable funding model for social care, supported by a diverse, vibrant and stable market; and
- greater security for all – for those born or developing a care need early in life and for those entering old age who do not know what their future care needs may be.

All of this proved to be yet another false policy dawn. Despite being originally slated for publication in the summer of 2017, five deadlines came and went, after which little was heard of it while political attention struggled to cope with the Brexit agenda. In the 2019 general election campaign, the Labour Party chose to make much of its commitment to reforming adult social care, pledging the provision of free personal care, the resumption of public sector provision and the 'ethical commissioning' of services and support. The Conservative Party manifesto, by contrast, made no mention of the missing Green Paper and made no other specific commitments. Nevertheless, when Boris Johnson became Prime Minister, he focused on adult social care in his very first speech, saying:

> 'My job is to protect you or your parents or grandparents from the fear of having to sell your home to pay for the costs of care and so I am announcing now – on the steps of Downing Street – that we will fix the crisis in social care once and for all with a clear plan we have prepared to give every older person the dignity and security they deserve.'

By this point, all mention of the Green Paper had vanished and the attention seemed to be back on the narrower matter of funding long-term care and focused entirely on older people. There was now no mention of social care for other adults or of any of the broader principles identified by Jeremy Hunt, who had left office by then. Although Johnson referred to 'a clear plan we have prepared', there was no indication of what this plan might be, when it would be put into effect or if it even existed. Indeed, when, within a few weeks, it was announced that 'cross-party talks' were required to try to forge a new consensus on the matter, a sense of déjà vu became overwhelming.

As noted earlier, the political focus is firmly on the position of older people and what contribution to their care costs is equitable. This risks ignoring the situation of younger adults needing adult social care and support – largely people with learning disabilities, mental health problems and other complex needs. This is a growing area of need: the proportion of younger adults reporting a disability increased from 14 per cent in 2007/08 to 18 per cent in 2017/18, while the number of people with severe learning disabilities is projected to rise by 34 per cent between 2017 and 2027 (Idriss et al, 2020). In terms of expenditure, this age group currently accounts for around half of all local authority spending on adult social care.

Although still resembling a policy graveyard, all of this suggests that adult social care – its funding, organisation, structure and delivery – is at least rising up the political agenda. It has certainly been on a tortuous journey. Over a 70-year period, it has moved from being a small and obscure responsibility of local councils to being a multi-billion pound market for investors, a major employer of staff, a massive challenge for local government commissioning and a financial calamity for many of those who depend upon services and support. The nature of the sector has changed hugely from a public ownership model to a 'quasi-market' model – one in which much of the commissioning or purchasing of services and support is still largely within the remit of the public sector but provision is largely undertaken by private companies. Alongside this, the requirement to draw upon savings and capital assets has resulted in a massive number of 'self-funders' – individuals who purchase their own support in this new care market. Although not the only policy domain to be shaped by such a retreat from state provision, it was probably the first to be so comprehensively reshaped.

This metamorphosis from state to market has been 40 years in the making: the foundations were securely put in place over two key decades – the 1980s and 1990s – and the consequences have been played out in the first two decades of the 21st century. With the third decade of the 21st century getting under way, it might be tempting to see much of this as being of little more than historical interest. That would be a mistake. What the longer-term perspective in this book offers is the opportunity to: understand the advantages and disadvantages of what might be loosely termed a 'neoliberal' model of public policy; identify more carefully the objectives and expectations of the shift; consider the extent to which these have been fulfilled; and consider options going ahead. In understanding more about the fortunes of adult social care, it is also possible to raise broader issues that can help to inform the debate in other policy domains that are currently on a similar trajectory of 'marketisation'.

The title of the book encapsulates the contours of the debate – the ways in which those who require some form of care and support are variously depicted as clients, consumers or citizens, each implying very different relationships between the state, professionals, families, communities and individuals. This is far from being a settled debate. On 14 January 2020, Prime Minister Boris Johnson was questioned about the reform of the sector during an interview on BBC Breakfast. His comments seemed to suggest the need to go back to first principles:

> 'It's a big thing and we've got to get it right because there's a lot of really quite important moral and social issues contained within it. Should taxpayers be paying for people who might be able to afford it? What is the relationship between families that you want to encourage? Should families be looking after their elderly relatives? All these are very complex questions.'

Notwithstanding this high degree of ongoing uncertainty, in broad terms, we can understand the post-war era between 1945 and 1980 as predominantly the era of a state-delivered service characterised by the importance of the professional–client relationship – indeed, this interaction was itself often identified as an end product. The post-1980 period can be characterised as one in which the inherently paternalistic nature of this relationship was challenged by 'consumerism', a model thought to be better equipped for meeting individual needs and preferences. Now, in the 2020s, there is renewed – if nascent – interest in ideas around community, co-production and citizenship. The debates swimming around underneath these concepts are the concern of this book, the rest of which is structured as follows:

- Chapter 1 describes and examines the pre-market era in 'social services': the Victorian interventions and their ongoing influence; the post-1945 era in which state provision was shaped by the National Assistance Act 1948; and the brief ascendancy of state-run provision in the wake of the 1968 Seebohm Report (Seebohm Committee, 1968) and the Local Authority Social Services Act 1970.
- Chapter 2 explores the emergence of 'neoliberalism' as the dominant approach to politics and policy in the 1980s, and the way in which this led to critiques of the state-run model of the 1970s. It charts the subsequent emergence of the market model based upon the split between the commissioning of services and their provision, and the growing acceptance of this as the new paradigm.
- Chapter 3 looks at dilemmas in commissioning. Now that the 'purchaser–provider split' is entrenched, what judgement can we make of how well commissioning has lived up to expectations?

How is the concept being understood and interpreted? What are its strengths and weaknesses?

- Chapter 4 explores dilemmas in provision. Has the market delivered the right sort of care where it is needed? Is it a robust model capable of meeting current and future demands? Is there a workforce available in the right numbers and with the right skills?
- Chapter 5 takes stock of the ongoing arguments about the relative merits and demerits of provision by the state or through the market. Where the market has defects, can these be remedied? Is a return to public sector provision feasible?
- Chapter 6 examines the crucial contexts of funding and administration. What scale of resources is needed to ensure that adult social care is able to meet anticipated need? How can local government be strengthened to fulfil its statutory functions?
- Chapter 7 develops a new framework for the commissioning of ethical care with several components: ethical business commissioning; commissioning local and small; commissioning personally; and commissioning for well-being.
- Chapter 8 looks at the impact of COVID-19 on adult social care. Was it a system able to withstand an emergency event? How was the position of the sector understood by politicians and policymakers? What lessons can be learned for the future?
- Chapter 9 returns to the issues of morals, markets and power. What is the most appropriate place for market principles in adult social care? How could ethical principles be put centre stage? How can change be supported and sustained?

Most of these issues have been considered in some way before and this book draws upon these existing insights and analyses. Commissions, parliamentary select committees, think tanks, academic researchers and others have examined almost every aspect. Organisations representing those who use services or have caring responsibilities have long pressed the case for better treatment, while those advising financial investors have pored over market trends. In addition, as noted earlier, political manifestos have made a multitude of pledges that subsequently fail to be delivered. In that sense, everything in this book is already out there somewhere. However, what has not been done is to bring all of this together into a coherent narrative that describes the changes, examines the problems and proposes some solutions. The aim of this volume is to fill precisely that gap.

1

Before the market

The institutional legacy

The adult social care services that are available today have evolved from the residual institutional provision that was made available to paupers of all ages under the Victorian Poor Law (Thane, 1996). Although the Poor Law was revoked to widespread acclaim by the National Assistance Act 1948, unlike other sectors (notably, health, housing and education), no comprehensive policy was introduced to replace it. The 1948 Act (Section 21) stated that it should be the duty of every local authority to set up a 'welfare department' to provide 'residential accommodation for persons who by reason of age, infirmity or any other circumstances are in need of care and attention which is not otherwise available to them'. Section 28 further empowered local authorities 'to promote the welfare of persons who were blind, deaf or dumb, and others who were substantially and permanently handicapped by illness, injury or congenital deformity'.

These obligations to offer institutional care constituted a clear reflection of Victorian policy solutions. It still remained ultra vires for local authorities to develop preventive services like meals-on-wheels, chiropody, laundry, visiting schemes or counselling – these were viewed as 'extras' and therefore the domain of the voluntary sector (Parker, 1965). Changes to this situation took place slowly. The National Assistance (Amendment) Act 1962 for the first time allowed local authorities to provide meal services directly, as opposed to making grants available to the third sector. The Health Services and Public Health Act 1968 further afforded councils a general power to promote the welfare of older people, while a private members bill introduced by Alf Morris MP resulted in the Chronically Sick and Disabled Persons Act 1970, which was designed to compel local authorities to develop comprehensive welfare and support services for disabled people (Means et al, 2002).

These powers to develop preventive services were not matched by the allocation of additional resources, leaving local authority welfare departments small and marginalised. Even the main remit of these departments – residential care – was not undertaken particularly well.

In the case of older people, Townsend (1964) noted a lack of investment across all welfare institutions caring for older people. In 1949, 40,000 residents were housed in former workhouses, and by 1960, the figure was still 35,000. Where local councils drew up development plans, these were often curtailed by central government restrictions on capital expenditure, and although new and smaller homes did open in the 1950s and 1960s, these were insufficient to allow the closure of existing capacity.

A similar situation applied to provision for working-age adults; a detailed survey by Miller and Gwynne (1972) found inadequate 'warehoused' residential care being offered as the only option for an entire lifespan. Meanwhile, the legacy of large asylums continued to dominate provision for many people with mental health problems and learning disabilities. Public funding had poured into asylum construction between 1800 and 1900 as Victorians placed faith in bricks-and-mortar solutions to social problems. These buildings were designed to be majestic, therapeutic and durable, and efforts to reduce their role had only limited effect as late as the 1970s (Jones, 1972).

The winds of change

The political and policy landscape began to change in many ways by the mid-1960s. In his magisterial review of the post-war welfare state, Timmins (1995: 215) notes:

> It was the start of the high noon for the high priests of planning – the apogee of a two-decade stretch in which both economic and welfare state problems were seen to be susceptible to the answers of planning and agreement....
> It was a heyday for Royal Commissions and government inquiries, for faith in the views of experts, the whole enterprise undertaken with the certainty that solutions were there if only one could think of them.

Although largely driven by the Labour governments of 1964–70, this approach had roots in the late 1950s under a Conservative government. In particular, Enoch Powell, the Health Minister, launched his 1962 Hospital Plan. This foresaw a closure programme for large mental health and (in the vernacular of the time) 'mental handicap' hospitals, and their replacement by a network of community services. The fact that this goal has not yet been fully achieved even in 2020 should not deflect from the principle behind Powell's plan, which – given the significance of the Victorian legacy – was far-sighted.

In the case of social care (for both children and adults), the real catalyst for change was the report of the Seebohm Committee (1968). The committee was set up in 1965 by the Home Secretary, the Secretary of State for Education and Science, the Minister of Housing and Local Government, and the Minister of Health. This multiple political commitment was an achievement in itself given the tradition of working in silo departments. Its purpose was to 'review the organisation and responsibilities of the local authority personal social services in England and Wales, and to consider what changes are desirable to secure an effective family service'. The report was critical of the fragmented nature of existing services, arguing that this was producing separate spheres of responsibility with neglected areas between – a critique that has since been echoed down the decades.

The view of the committee was that social workers should cease concentrating on a series of isolated issues (mental health, physical disability, homelessness and so on) and should instead concentrate on helping families, that is, to be family-oriented rather than problem-oriented. Working within a strengthened public sector organisation was seen as key to promoting this vision. It was accordingly recommended that new unified social services departments be created. These were to be large local authority institutions with a correspondingly strong committee structure, and were expected to be chaired by a powerful local councillor who could embed and develop the model. Their duties were to incorporate children's and welfare services, plus some of the services then provided by local health, education and housing departments. This was all a far cry from the small children's departments and weak welfare departments ushered in after the Second World War.

Moreover, this shift was to be cultural, not simply organisational. In contrast to the deterrence culture of the Poor Law, one of the key reasons for the changes was to encourage people in need to use services. Here was a model aiming at: better detection of need and greater encouragement to seek help; attracting more resources and using them more efficiently; and planning more systematically for the future (Hallett, 1982). In a vision that would not be out of place in modern conceptions of co-production and citizenship, the committee argued for change 'not simply in terms of organisation but as embodying a wider conception of social services directed to the wellbeing of the whole of the community and not only the social casualties, and seeing the community it serves as the basis of its authority, resources and effectiveness' (Seebohm Committee, 1968: 147). The Seebohm blueprint only just made it onto the statute book. The last act of the Labour government in 1970 prior to calling a general election (which it would lose) was to gain royal assent on the day Parliament was dissolved. The Local Authority Social Services Act 1970, implementing the basis of the report, went ahead. It was, said Timmins (1995: 231), 'a grand and comprehensive vision ... a great leap forward for the personal social services'.

The terminology of the time is relevant here – the terms 'personal social services' and 'social services department' were used, rather than the now universal 'adult social care'. Even as late as 1999, a glossary of terms published by the Royal Commission on Long Term Care listed neither 'social care' nor 'adult social care' as being in use. Indeed, Smith et al (2019) find the term first being used in a relatively obscure guidance document on eligibility published in 2003 (Department of Health, 2003). The changing terminology is consistent with wider shifts around the concepts of client, consumer and citizen (Mayer and Timms, 1970).

The emerging critique

The Seebohm model was based upon faith in the capacity of bureaucracies to organise and plan, and in the ability of professionals to understand and resolve the problems of individuals and communities. It was a model driving other parts of the post-war welfare state in housing, education, healthcare and social security. In adult social care, as elsewhere, there was an assumption of a strong state (central or local) planning, funding, employing and providing support on the back of a shared endeavour. It was also, in the first few years, a well-funded model, with investment going into residential care, day care, fieldwork and professional training.

As with much else, the visit of the International Monetary Fund in 1976 to bail out the Labour government from a financial crisis led to the first of many funding problems for the sector (Jones, 2020). It also coincided with other ideological and social trends in such a way that the Seebohm model was undermined within only a few short years. Before the decade was out, disaffection was focused upon the structure and hierarchical nature of social services departments, a critique reflected in the phrase 'Seebohm factories' (Simpkin, 1979). In doing so, the space began to be created for a totally different approach rooted in the efficacy of markets driven by consumer power and preference.

If the mid-1960s was the high point of faith in expertise and planning, then the mid-1970s was the beginning of the claims for a totally different world view, one often encapsulated by the term 'neoliberalism'. The concept is slippery (Johnson, 2014) but rooted in the view that: the state is inherently inefficient when compared with markets; the welfare state has become too large to be manageable; and governments should concentrate on making strategic policy decisions rather than become involved with the direct delivery of services.

Within this world view, competition is seen as the defining characteristic of human relations and citizens are accordingly redefined as consumers – as individuals whose democratic choices are best exercised by buying and selling. Where many 'consumers' have insufficient funds to buy their own services, as in the case of adult social care, then the state should seek to do that on their behalf by 'shaping the market' in a way that ensures support is available that meets their needs (Le Grand, 2009). Brown and Jacobs (2008) pithily describe the core teachings of this approach in terms of 'five pathologies':

- *Government mainly fails*: public policies seem not to achieve much towards fulfilling their announced goals.
- *Government is incompetent*: we do not know the relationship between the public policies we adopt and the effects these policies were designed to achieve.
- *Government means capture*: interest groups intent on maximising their own interests 'acquire policies'.
- *Government abridges freedom*: agreement by political decisions entails a one-size-fits-all conformity at the expense of individuals, who are seen as better equipped to collect and process information and reach decisions.
- *Government only gets worse*: once in place, public agencies become self-governing bodies run by self-serving careerists.

This approach requires a 'shrinking state' (Lobao et al, 2018) – an erosion of the state from its customary intervention in regulating economic growth and promoting redistribution, and the overall weakening of the state as an institution in local and regional affairs. The role of the state in many capitalist countries came under attack in the 1980s, when it was accused of allocating resources inefficiently and crowding out resources that could have been put to better use by the private sector. This led to attempts to diminish the role of the state by means of: reductions in public expenditure; the privatisation of public assets; the introduction of markets or 'quasi-markets' into the public sector; reducing taxation; and reducing labour market regulations. The election of a Conservative government led by Margaret Thatcher in

1979 catalysed these ideas and weakened the notion that the state could act as a benign instrument for securing social policy goals (Deakin, 1994). With bureaucratic decision-making coming under attack, the consequences for the newly created social services departments were enormous, being increasingly portrayed as offering a top-down, 'take it or leave it' model of care that marginalised service users and carers.

Front-line professionals were seen as complicit in this – a complete change from the slow progress towards professional status that had rested upon the place of professional insight into the needs of their clients. This position stemmed from the casework lineage of the Charity Organisation Society from the 1860s onward (Humphreys, 2001) and the growing emphasis on the significance of 'the relationship' between professional and client. The American doyen of casework Florence Hollis (1948: 5) described the caseworker as one who 'assists families and individuals in developing both the capacity and opportunity to lead personally satisfying and socially useful lives'. In Britain, the social work profession was hugely influenced by similar ideas from Eileen Younghusband (1965). This approach came to be seen as a means of supporting individuals to adjust to, and cope with, their adverse circumstances.

Others were beginning to take a different view. In a memorable assault on the notion of the 'professional–client relationship' in the late 1950s, the sociologist Barbara Wootton (1959: 5) argued that, if taken at face value, prevalent definitions of 'social casework' 'involved claims to powers which verge upon omniscience and omnipotence'. She noted the significance of the psychoanalytical influence, with the emphasis on the relationship between the social worker and those who either seek aid or have it thrust upon them, and the way 'the relationship' had become the central theme in the literature on social work practice. For Wootton (1959: 277), this had led to a practice whereby social workers 'refused to accept at face value the emergencies which caused people to seek aid', with moral judgements concealed in what appeared to be the neutral language of science.

More significantly, this critique was later taken up by some of those in receipt of care and support. This resulted in a series of struggles by different user movements about relations of domination and dependency that challenged both policy and practice, especially the normative exercise of professional power over service users (Clarke, 2006). The notion of 'need' is central to this discourse, with user movements being highly critical of professional claims to expertise about the nature of people's needs. The year 1981 was the International Year of Disabled People and saw the establishment of the increasingly influential British Council of Organisations of Disabled People, which, by 2002, comprised 130 independent organisations representing over 400,000 disabled people. This was an important point in the struggle for power between organisations *of* disabled people and organisations *for* them.

The social model of disability (Campbell and Oliver, 1996) was highly critical of previous attempts to individualise and 'medicalise' disability in ways that reduce it to matters of functional limitation. Rather, it was argued that society disables people, for example, through segregated education, inadequate access to the labour market and standardised care packages. Direct payments emerged from this struggle as a way of attempting to deliver autonomy and choice to service users – the Community Care (Direct Payments) Act 1996 gave physically disabled people and people with learning difficulties (below the age of 65) the possibility of receiving a payment to arrange their own care services. The Act arose from a private members bill advocated by the British Council of Organisations of Disabled People and the Independent Living Movement, but at this stage, it was only a permissive power with no guarantee of local availability.

At the same time, there were radical forces at work within the social work profession itself, including influential left-wing writers such as Bailey and Brake (1975) and Corrigan and Leonard (1978). Whereas Wootton identified a valuable role for social workers as expert 'navigators' through the maze of welfare services, the radical social work school was more concerned to locate the oppression of individuals in the context of social and economic structures. It criticised the capitalist system and traditional social work, seeing the true role of social work as being to change capitalist society and eliminate its 'pathologising' approach to individuals needing help.

In more practical terms, the relatively short-lived monthly social work magazine *Case Con* complemented the academic development of radical social work in the early 1970s. Alongside this, from 1970 to 1978, the British government funded 12 community development projects (CDPs) in some of the most impoverished neighbourhoods in England, Scotland and Wales. These were given resources to hire researchers and community workers to work alongside community residents towards the goal of ameliorating deleterious local conditions. By 1978, all 12 projects had been shut down amid a great deal of political acrimony from those unhappy with their radical stance (Loney, 1981).

Although coming from starkly different political positions, the forces of neoliberalism, the disabled people's movement and the radical social work model coalesced in their critique of the traditional post-war welfare state model espoused by the Seebohm reforms. Given the political dominance of reforming right-wing Conservative governments from 1979 to 1997, followed by centrist 'New Labour' regimes, the radical social work model all but vanished. While the disabled people's movement could point to some successes – albeit contested – with direct payments and their successor 'personal budgets', the real victor was the neoliberal school of thought. The 1980s saw the emergence and establishment of these ideas in public policy in general, and in adult social care in particular. Such developments are the focus of Chapter 2.

Chapter summary

Adult social care has its roots in a residual means-tested approach to support that was the hallmark of Victorian social policy. Although the post-war welfare state of the 1940s led to comprehensive and universal strategies for health, education, housing and social security, this was not the case with adult social care, which stuck to a minimalist model. The report of the Seebohm Committee (1968), followed by the Local Authority Social Services Act 1970, led to a brief period of local state renaissance for the sector; however, by the 1980s, this bureaucratic-professional model was coming under attack from some service users and from increasingly influential neoliberal thinkers. The seeds had been sown for a new approach to the sector rooted in markets, competition and choice.

2

The emergence and consolidation of the market

Introduction

Developments in adult social care in the 1980s did not emerge in isolation from wider policies in the public realm. Although the public sector has always bought goods and services from the private sector, the influence of neoliberal ideas in the 1980s opened up the debate on whether this should go further than hitherto. In the 1979 Conservative government's first legislative programme, the principle of compulsory competitive tendering for building work was introduced by the Planning and Local Government Act 1980; this principle was later extended to most local authority direct labour work under the Local Government Act 1988. In the same year, the Housing Reform Act encouraged council tenants to 'opt out' of local authority control by choosing new landlords (termed 'housing action trusts') in the not-for-profit sector. Meanwhile, changes in the NHS were not dissimilar, with organisational responsibility for funding and managing service delivery separated through a 'purchaser–provider split'.

Underpinning these ideas was the emergent concept of 'new public management' (Hood, 1995). This also proposed a quasi-market structure, whereby public and private service providers competed with each other in an attempt to provide better and faster services. Other core themes included: a strong focus on financial control, value for money and increasing efficiency; introducing audits at both financial and professional levels to review performance; greater customer orientation and responsiveness; increasing the scope of roles played by non-public sector providers; deregulating the labour market; discouraging the self-regulatory power of professionals; and handing over power from management to individuals. If neoliberalism provided the ideological framework, new public management offered the means of delivery.

In the social care context, a key landmark was the speech in 1984 by the then Secretary of State for Health, Norman Fowler (1984), extolling the virtues of the 'enabling role' of local government. He suggested that social services departments should switch their focus from the direct provision of care to the funding and facilitation of the delivery of care. Accordingly, he set out three roles for social services departments and the wider local council remit:

- a comprehensive strategic view of all available sources of care;
- a recognition that social services were only part of the local pattern; and
- a recognition that social services should support and promote the fullest possible participation of the other different sources of care that exist or can be called into being.

The concept of the 'purchaser–provider' split had already been proposed in relation to the delivery of healthcare and applying the idea to social services was quickly seized upon by the Thatcher government. Responsibility for the planning and commissioning of services was to be separated from the delivery of services: the purchaser would specify what was required and secure the most effective and efficient way to deliver the service from a range of competing providers.

All of these developments show the influence of neoliberal critiques of public bureaucracies as self-interested, budget-maximising agencies protected from competitive forces. The government now spends £284 billion a year on buying goods and services from external suppliers (IFG Consulting, 2018), amounting to around a third of all public expenditure. This money is spent on everything from goods such as stationery and medicine, through to the construction of schools and roads, the daily delivery of back-office functions such as information technology and human resources, and the provision of front-line services such as probation and parts of the NHS. However, of all social policy domains, it is adult social care where the penetration of the market model has been quickest and deepest. The way in which this occurred has shaped the nature of service delivery to this day.

1980s: the emergent market

The chronological narrative behind the opening up of the market in adult social care in the 1980s is still shrouded in some uncertainty. The lever for change consisted of a seemingly insignificant change in the financial assessment of older people on low incomes in relation to their potential residence in private care homes. Before 1980, the central government assistance authority for those on subsistence income (the Supplementary Benefits Commission) was generally unwilling to financially support people in the private sector. However, in a little-noticed change, the rules were then relaxed and local social security office managers were given considerable discretion to subsidise charges in private care homes through means-tested benefit payments.

These taxation-funded payments were subsequently made available nationwide to all who passed an income- and asset-based means test. Payments covered board, lodging and personal expense costs but were only payable to those in private residential care homes as opposed to those run by local councils or the third sector. Moreover, there was initially no cap whatsoever on the costs attached to these payments – social security payments met whatever fees were being charged to residents. Understandably, this led to a rapid expansion in private sector homes and accompanying concerns about the cost to the public purse. By 1983, it became necessary to introduce national limits on payable fees, though these were still set at a much higher rate than those that had prevailed before 1980, when commercial home charges were rarely fully met. The subsequent dramatic growth in private sector care homes was then extended to nursing homes that were doing work previously considered to be the domain of the NHS; a special high social assistance rate was allowed for these.

To this day, it is unclear whether all of this was a policy accident or a policy design, but given that the impetus came from obscure and unheralded changes in the social security system (rather than directly from within adult social care), it seems to be more a matter of policy happenstance than strategic vision. Hardy and Wistow (2000) certainly took the view that the dramatic growth in social security support to the independent sector as a whole was unplanned, and took place despite a series of attempts to check its growth. The figures are striking. In December 1979, supplementary benefit paid to support individuals in residential and nursing home care provided by the independent sector amounted to £10 million (12,000 claimants). By May 1991, this had increased to £1,872 million and 231,000 claimants; by May 1993, the figures were £2,480 million and 270,000 claimants (House of Commons Social Security Committee, 1991). The privatisation revolution in adult social care was up and running.

Whatever the policy genesis, it had immediate effects on other sectors and services. The first casualty was non-residential support; with no equivalent social security support for domiciliary care, the effect was to seriously constrain its development. The second casualty was residential care provided by local authorities; council-funded residential care spending was flat during this period as local authorities happily took advantage of the opportunity to shift costs from the ratepayer to the taxpayer. Finally, it encouraged the NHS to take the opportunity to divest itself of geriatric hospital beds (free at the point of use) and move these into the means-tested sector of adult social care. All of these shifts – considered to be minor or smartly opportunistic at the time – have had massive subsequent consequences.

1990s: the regulated market

The social security subsidy soon became financially unsustainable and the Thatcher government of the 1980s began to cast around for solutions in terms of financial control and service delivery. An important critique of the impact of the subsidy on service delivery came in an influential report from the Audit Commission (1986), which highlighted the failure to develop community-based provision at the expense of residential care. It identified a pattern of slow and uneven progress in developing community-based services, being caused by:

- disincentives for local authorities to invest in community care stemming from a mismatch between policy objectives and funding systems;
- a lack of bridging finance to support the shift from hospitals to care in the community;
- perverse incentives from an income support system that supported care in residential and nursing homes but not in other settings;
- organisational fragmentation and confusion in the responsibilities of agencies at all levels; and
- staffing problems resulting from the absence of workforce planning and effective staff training for community care.

It would be harsh to argue that these problems had arisen directly as a result of the Seebohm reforms – indeed, most of them are still problematic today. The government's response was to commission a high-level review led by a trusted business ally of the Prime Minister, Sir Roy Griffiths. His subsequent report (Griffiths, 1988) effectively killed off the fledgling Seebohm model of state planning, funding and delivery of local services. Griffiths sought to eliminate the perverse incentive towards residential care by recommending that a unified community care budget be allocated to local social services authorities in the form of a specific grant (the Special Transitional Grant), principally composed of resources transferred from the social security system. However, at the same time, he proposed a major recasting of the role of local authorities so that they would function as the designers, organisers and purchasers of non-healthcare services, and not primarily as direct providers. Moreover, he wanted them to be making the maximum possible use of voluntary and private sector bodies in order to widen consumer choice, stimulate innovation and encourage efficiency. The ideas in Norman Fowler's (1984) speech were coming to fruition.

These proposals represented something of a dilemma for the Thatcher government. While it urgently needed to control the growth of social security expenditure on adult social care, it was reluctant to give further powers to local authorities, not least because most of them were under the control of other political parties. Under the terms of the Local Government Act 1985, the government had already taken steps to abolish the six county councils of the metropolitan counties that had been set up in 1974, along with the Greater London Council that had been established in 1965. All were seen as rivalrous sources of political power and the government had no wish to strengthen the powers of the remaining local councils. The inability to find an alternative solution explained the long delay between the publication of the Griffiths Report in 1988 and subsequent steps to implement its recommendations.

In the end, local authorities *were* given control of the social security budget but at the price of dismantling their Seebohm inheritance. The ensuing 1989 White Paper (Department of Health, 1989) proposed that local authority social services departments should take on responsibility for assessing the needs of, and purchasing care for, those who would previously have looked to the social security system to finance their care. These ideas then became the basis of the NHS and Community Care Act 1990, which was implemented in stages over the next three years. The White Paper's underlying purpose was described as one of 'promoting choice and independence', a purpose that was reflected in six key objectives:

- promoting the development of domiciliary, day and respite services to enable people to live in their own homes wherever feasible and sensible;
- ensuring that service providers make practical support for carers a high priority;
- making proper assessment of need and good case management the cornerstone of high-quality care;
- promoting the development of a flourishing independent sector alongside good-quality public services;

- clarifying the responsibilities of agencies, thereby making it easier to hold them to account for their performance; and
- securing better value for taxpayers' money by introducing a new funding structure for social care.

Some 30 years later, it would be a generous policy analyst who felt able to conclude that any of these objectives had been achieved – Chapters 3 and 4 will consider this further.

Importantly, local authorities were not at liberty to use this fresh funding stream as they thought fit; the neoliberal sting lay in the tail. First, to ensure that this money was used to develop the non-statutory sectors, it was stipulated that 85 per cent of the new funding was to be used *only* in those sectors, thereby effectively blocking the expansion of statutory provision. Second, new national standards for care homes concerning space and facilities were introduced. These would have required the upgrading of most local authority homes but centrally imposed restrictions on local authority capital borrowing and expenditure made it impossible for them to be upgraded to these standards. In effect, the first of these measures incentivised investment in the non-statutory sector while the second deterred investment in the statutory sector. By the simple route of pulling levers of resource allocation, the door was suddenly opened to the widespread privatisation of all adult social care.

This shift also had enormous implications for front-line practitioners. The Griffiths Report made no mention of social work, but the implications for social work practice were profound as they became responsible for assessing need and orchestrating packages of care, rather than directly delivering care. The counselling role stemming from the casework tradition and supported by the earlier Barclay Inquiry into the roles and tasks of social work (Barclay, 1982) was further eroded, as was the Seebohm Report's emphasis on community development and community social work.

The Barclay Report was the end result of a two-year inquiry into the roles and tasks of social workers in England and Wales. It was commissioned by the Secretary of State for Social Services in the first Thatcher government and produced by a working party convened by the National Institute for Social Work, chaired by Sir Peter Barclay. The report identified three main sets of assumptions about the relationship between the state and its citizens: the 'safety-net approach' (which values informal networks and minimal state provision); the 'welfare state approach' (the post-war idea of comprehensive services and citizens having a right to these); and the 'community approach' (which believes that people have the potential to care for each other if power is devolved to them and that the social worker's role is then to support these informal networks and develop them where they were weak).

The majority of committee members supported the third approach, highlighting the value of community social work. They called for more emphasis on community engagement, with a new role for social workers as brokers of resources, working with informal carers and voluntary organisations to support individual service users as citizens. The report's recommendations were largely ignored by the Thatcher government, though some local authorities did, for a time, introduce 'patch-based' approaches in response to the Barclay Report (Hadley and Hatch, 1981). However, the changes ushered in by the NHS and Community Care Act 1990 could not have been more different to the vision of the Barclay Report.

The 1990 Act introduced the seemingly innocuous notion of 'case management' (soon rebadged as 'care management') to describe this new role but it soon became evident that assessments were being used as a mechanism for prioritising needs and restricting access to services for all but those deemed most at risk of harm (Rummery and Glendinning, 2000). Carey (2015) argues that these changes to the social work role promoted inconsistent and unreliable services, the development of superficial relations with users and carers, and the loss of belonging and fractured identities of social care employees. All of this contributed to a cultural shift away from the established values of social work and social care, and towards the promotion of market mechanisms. The development of non-statutory service providers was itself seen as the guarantor of 'consumer benefits' by way of widening choice, promoting innovation and meeting individual needs. On the basis of this belief, there was therefore little need for a relationship between a social worker and a service user other than to assess eligibility for access to support and to help to construct a care package if requested.

These reforms were designed to achieve the most far-reaching and complex changes in the funding, organisation and delivery of social care services since the creation of the post-war welfare state. The task was (and remains) technically and politically demanding: technically because it requires substantial development of skills in the areas of needs identification, service specification, quality assurance and market shaping; and politically in that it requires a shift from the traditional local authority culture of civic pride in provision, to a less tangible role in helping to secure outcomes for users and carers. Local authorities were called upon to take over the operation of established local social care markets and to create a largely new market structure capable of meeting a set of challenging policy objectives in the long run. The cash-limited funding transferred to councils incentivised them to tighten eligibility criteria for access to support, ushering in a shift from a purely financial means test to one that also required an assessment of need. This regime of tighter eligibility criteria, caps on fee rates and tougher regulation on physical standards set in train a trend that continues to this day.

Although (as will be explored later) it is now routine to view local authorities as labouring under impossible circumstances, it is important to recount that at this stage in the narrative, opposition to the new paradigm was muted. This could have been down to a combination of relief at the acquisition of a fresh income stream allied to a failure to think through the longer-term consequences of this acquiescence. In time, the tight budgetary controls exercised at the centre, combined with an unfunded transfer of responsibilities from the NHS, would prove to be crippling burdens.

Meanwhile, notions of choice, independence, enabling and needs-led care planning held a superficial attraction for all parties. Local authorities chose to feel reassured by talk of a 'level playing field' that seemed to assure ongoing roles in provision for the statutory, voluntary and private sectors. Ideology and rhetoric combined with minimal evidence and muted resistance to bring about this momentous policy shift. There was also little wider party-political resistance or even interest – the reforms were introduced by a Conservative government but the 1992 Labour Party manifesto supported the general thrust of the changes and did not propose a reassertion of public sector dominance. Indeed, despite the huge policy significance of the shift to a market model, it had been the subject of relatively little debate as an idea.

The consolidated market

Once the nature and significance of the 1990 Act became clearer, there was some initial resistance on the part of those local authorities with a strong tradition of publicly provided services. This resistance was captured at the time in two studies of around 25 local authorities by Wistow et al (1994, 1996). The first study (undertaken between 1990 and 1992) found that the sites studied had made little progress on clarifying their position in relation to the changes, maybe hoping the consequences would pass them by or be only marginal in nature. In the follow-up study in the same authorities (based on 1993 data), the researchers reported greater understanding and awareness but still a reluctance to fully expose their in-house services to unprotected competition from the private and voluntary sectors in the belief that this would undermine existing high-quality provision.

In the first of these two studies, the research team identified ten 'provider options' in this post-1990 Act scenario, which they labelled A through J:

A. continuing local authority provision as organised in 1991 with no planned changes to the management, funding or regulation of activities;
B. continuing local authority provision with the reorganisation of the social services department along the lines of a purchaser–provider split of some kind and to some degree;
C. management or staff buyouts of some local authority services;
D. floating off some services to not-for-profit trusts, allowing the authority to retain some degree of control;
E. selling services, perhaps at a nominal price, to voluntary organisations that act independently of the authority except for any service agreements or contracts;
F. selling services to private (for-profit) agencies that act independently of the authority except for any service agreements or contracts;
G. encouraging voluntary or not-for-profit organisations setting up new services;
H. encouraging private (for-profit) agencies setting up new services;
I. considering health authorities as potential providers of some social care services; and
J. bringing NHS trusts into the supply picture.

The researchers found mixed responses from across social services authorities, often dependent upon political control and outlook. Most Labour-controlled authorities preferred options D and E, strongly preferred E to F, and were unhappy with H. Most Conservative-controlled authorities supported option G, had practical rather than ideological reservations about H and liked the idea of E and F. Underpinning all of these variations was near-universal anxiety about resources, pride in their own previous service provision and doubts about the potential of alternative sources of provision.

In their follow-up study, the research team found some evidence of change but also continuing reservations about the viability of the mission. In a significant (but small) minority, a complete divestment of provision was considered to be feasible; however, the majority of authorities reported their preferred supply development option to be the establishment of voluntary sector providers. On the one hand, there was said to be evidence of optimism about meeting the objectives of the White Paper by market mechanisms. On the other hand, there was also anxiety about the operation of social care markets – an anxiety that formed part of a wider concern that authorities needed to learn to manage the market, both to avoid its collapse and to influence its emerging shape. These concerns could certainly be said to be prescient.

At that time, not all private sector providers were identified as 'profit maximisers'; many were small, local 'family' businesses, often run by people who had been previously employed by local councils. For them, professional goals could be ranked even more highly than commercial ones. However, the larger private sector organisations were more likely to prioritise profit maximisation – a trend that continues to this day. Concerns about the future were not confined to the statutory sector. The voluntary sector too began to express fears about losing autonomy and flexibility, and about compromising their advocacy and campaigning roles. Smaller groups in particular were concerned about the demands of bidding and fulfilling contracts (Taylor et al, 1995) – yet another concern that has continued to this day.

Part of the reason for the cautious welcome by local authorities to the introduction of market mechanisms was that they interpreted the requirements in different ways. Rather than looking upon the shift as a strict neoclassical model, it was possible to imbue it with less challenging strictures. Wistow et al (1994) found the new 'enabling' role being invested with three different meanings:

- *Enabling as personal development*: this focuses upon the enabling of individual users and carers to achieve improvements in their well-being and to participate in 'ordinary' lifestyles. It implied working to maximise the potential of individuals, and to enable them to influence the design and delivery of services to secure that end. All parties could subscribe to this concept while holding different views about how it could best be accomplished.
- *Enabling as community development*: this had a stronger focus on collective action. It stressed the mobilisation and support of community-based resources, especially those of the informal and local voluntary sectors. It suggested a role for social services authorities based less upon the direct provision of their own services and more on shaping and influencing the wider range of resources available within local communities. This interpretation was consistent with the community social work tradition and could be traced back to the Seebohm Report.

- *Enabling as market development*: here the role of social services departments was to be true to the principles of marketisation and to create and manage the mixed economy of care. This was the least popular interpretation. The authors could only find three out of 25 local authorities as enthusiasts for this model – a reluctance rooted in the view that social care was different in kind from other public services and ill suited to a market model.

The established market

The difficulty with the various local understandings of what a market in adult social care might look like was that the least popular interpretation was precisely the one incentivised by the 1990 Act and its accompanying regulation and guidance. Wishful thinking would not be enough to prevent this version from spreading. There were no further detailed studies of the emerging market in the rest of that decade, but it is clear that despite the initial reluctance and suspicion on the part of the statutory and voluntary sectors, the model evolved rapidly.

In considering this, it is important to be clear that the provision of adult social care had never been an *entirely* public sector realm. Nevertheless, the shift in sectoral provision on the back of the market-based reforms produced startling changes within less than a decade. Tables 1 and 2, both adapted from the 1998 annual state of the market surveys from LaingBuisson (1998), show how much the position changed in a short space of time for care home provision and home care provision, respectively.

This trend has continued unabated: a dramatic fall in statutory provision, a modest increase (at best) in third sector provision and a rapid increase in private sector provision. This situation is far from consistent with the objective identified in the 1989 White Paper of promoting the development of a flourishing independent sector alongside good quality public services. Rather, the 'level playing field' turned out to be a euphemism for private sector domination that has continued to this day. By March 2018, of 464,000 places in residential care homes and NHS long-stay hospitals, 81 per cent were operated by private for-profit providers, 13 per cent by not-for-profit providers and only 6 per cent by statutory sector providers, either local authority or NHS. In the case of home care, 98 per cent of English council-funded home care hours were outsourced to independent sector providers, mostly for-profit companies (LaingBuisson, 2018b).

Within this shift in sectoral provision, there has also been a trend towards larger provider groups at the expense of smaller ones. The

Table 1: Residential home care for elderly, chronically ill and physically disabled people, market share by sector, UK 1970–98 (%)

Year	Local authority	Private sector	Voluntary sector
1970	63	14	23
1975	66	13	21
1980	63	17	20
1985	51	32	17
1990	39	48	13
1991	37	50	13
1992	33	52	15
1993	30	53	17
1994	28	54	18
1995	26	55	19
1996	25	56	19
1997	23	59	18
1998	22	61	17

Source: LaingBuisson (1998)

Table 2: Local authority-purchased home care, market share by sector, 1992–97 (%)

Year	Local authority	Private sector	Voluntary sector
1992	98	2	0.4
1993	95	4	1
1994	81	16	3
1995	71	26	3
1996	64	32	3.4
1997	56	39	5

Source: LaingBuisson (1998)

introduction of a new regulatory regime with higher standards meant that many small providers had to close because they did not have access to the finance needed to bring their homes up to the required standard. This led to further growth in the share of the market owned by large investors. The large for-profit and not-for-profit groups were able to expand as they had access to the necessary finance, management and marketing expertise to do so. Smaller traditional owner/manager enterprises found it difficult to compete in this environment.

These changes are reflected in the focus of interest on the supply side over the decades. Writing of the position in 1991, Wistow et al (1994) identified four main provider sectors: the public sector, the voluntary sector, the private sector and the informal or household sector. It was noted that the boundaries between these sectors were blurred:

> Some private agencies disguise themselves as voluntary; some voluntary agencies behave in a manner fully consistent with maximisation of either profits or managers' salaries; and a growing number of public agencies are developing many of the trappings of commercial enterprises, or are establishing not-for-profit trusts to run certain services under contract. (Wistow et al, 1994: 32)

The major new entrant – the private sector – has been the most complex to understand, with a wide variety of different operators emerging. The Centre for Health and the Public Interest (CHPI, 2019) identified six main types of providers in operation during the initial market opening in the 1980s:

- *traditional owner/managers* (either new entrants with training in a caring profession or those involved in a career change)
- *coloniser chains* (over time, some of the smaller care home providers were transformed into such 'chains' by businesspeople seeking new areas of investment)
- *hotel and leisure interests* (companies with subsidiaries in gambling and brewing)
- *construction and property groups*
- *private for-profit healthcare groups*
- *private not-for-profit healthcare groups*

There has been a shift in the type of private provider in the intervening years. Around a fifth of provision is now in the hands of the five largest providers, four of which are owned by private equity firms. However, the provider sector is chiefly characterised by a multiplicity of competing providers, many of them small or medium-sized enterprises. The care home sector supports around 410,000 residents across 11,300 homes from 5,500 different providers (Competition and Markets Authority, 2017). The situation with domiciliary care is even more diverse, with almost 900,000 people receiving help from over 10,000 regulated providers (United Kingdom Home Care Association, 2016). This has all manner of implications for the ways in which the market can be shaped and regulated.

The paradigm shift from a state-planned, -funded and -provided service in adult social care to a market commodity is now almost complete. However, this is not a full market, but rather – as Le Grand (1991) dubbed it – a 'quasi-market' – one in which provision is effectively privatised but much of the purchasing (or commissioning) of care still lies with the public sector. This shift from direct service provision towards the use of market mechanisms in the public sector was described by Osborne and Gaebler (1992) as a change from governments 'rowing' to 'steering'.

Steering was seen as a radically new way of performing governance, whereby the government increased its contracting, commissioning and tendering to non-governmental organisations. However, as Carey et al (2020) point out, this does not equate to a self-regulating market. Rather – at the most basic level – governments are expected to create the conditions under which public sector quasi-markets can work effectively. For them, this means ensuring that: new providers can enter the market and grow; providers are competing actively and in desirable ways; providers are able to exit the market in an orderly way; those choosing services (whether service users or public officials choosing on their behalf) are motivated to make informed choices; and levels of funding are appropriate to achieve policy objectives. The extent to which the introduction of quasi-markets in adult social care has met these caveats is the focus of Chapters 3, 4 and 5.

Chapter summary

The 1980s saw growing interest on the part of governments in the outsourcing of service delivery to non-statutory agencies, with statutory authorities expected to focus upon the planning, commissioning and contracting roles. Other strategies – notably, those of 'new public management' – were designed to rein in professional discretion and empower 'consumers'. Adult social care became one of the first major policy domains to adopt this approach. Responsibility for the planning and commissioning of services was to be separated from the delivery of services: the purchaser would specify what was required and secure the most effective and efficient way to deliver the service from a range of competing providers.

The 1980s was the decade of an *emergent market* in adult social care. The lever for change consisted of a seemingly insignificant change in the financial assessment of older people on low incomes in relation to their residence in private care homes. Taxation-funded payments were made available nationwide to all who passed an income- and asset-based means test, and there was initially no cap on the costs attached to these payments. The subsequent dramatic growth in private sector homes was also extended to nursing homes.

The changes had immediate effects on other sectors and services. With no equivalent social security support for domiciliary care, the effect was to seriously constrain the development of the latter. Council-funded care home provision soon stalled as local authorities took advantage of the opportunity to shift costs from the ratepayer to the taxpayer. It also encouraged the NHS to take the opportunity to divest itself of geriatric hospital beds (free at the point of use) and move these into the means-tested sector.

The 1990s can be characterised as the decade of *market regulation* as attempts (with far-reaching consequences) were made to regulate the explosion of growth in the state-funded private care home market and change the shape of provision. An influential report from the Audit Commission highlighted the ways in which the subsidy for residential provision had led to a failure to develop community-based provision. Searching for a means of curbing the increase in expenditure, Prime Minister Margaret Thatcher appointed a trusted ally – Sir Roy Griffiths – to identify a solution. His report effectively killed off the fledgling Seebohm model of state planning, funding and delivery of local services. In line with the tenets of 'new public management', he proposed a major recasting of the role of local authorities so that they would function as the designers, organisers and purchasers of non-healthcare services, and not primarily as direct providers.

These changes also had enormous implications for front-line practitioners. The Griffiths Report made no mention of social work, but the implications for social work practice were profound as they now became responsible for assessing need and orchestrating packages of care, rather than directly delivering care. It soon became evident that assessments were being used as a mechanism for prioritising needs and restricting access to services for all but those deemed most at risk of harm. This required substantial development of skills in the areas of needs identification, service specification and quality assurance. This new regime of tighter eligibility criteria, caps on fee rates and tougher regulation of physical standards set in train a trend that continues to this day.

The emergent market was followed by the *consolidated market*. There was some initial resistance on the part of those local authorities with a strong tradition of publicly provided services. Underpinning this was near-universal anxiety about resources, pride in their own previous service provision and doubts about the potential of alternative sources of provision. This anxiety formed part of a wider concern that authorities needed to learn to manage the market, both to avoid its collapse and to influence its emerging shape. The voluntary sector too began to express fears about losing autonomy and flexibility, and about compromising their advocacy and campaigning roles.

Finally, the sector came to be characterised by the *established market*. Despite the initial reluctance and suspicion on the part of the statutory and voluntary sectors, the market model evolved rapidly. The shift in sectoral provision on the back of the market-based reforms produced startling changes within less than a decade. This trend has continued unabated: a dramatic fall in statutory provision, a modest increase (at best) in third sector provision and a rapid increase in private sector provision. Within this shift in sectoral provision, there has also been a trend towards larger provider groups at the expense of smaller ones. The large for-profit and not-for-profit groups were able to expand as they had access to the necessary finance, management and marketing expertise to do so. Smaller traditional owner/manager enterprises found it difficult to compete in this environment. The paradigm shift from a state-planned, -funded and -provided service in adult social care to a market commodity is now almost complete.

3

Dilemmas in the commissioning of adult social care

The nature of commissioning and outsourcing

In broad terms, 'commissioning' refers to the process of the planning and strategic purchasing of services. While there are many models available, they all fundamentally break down into four key areas:

- *analysis*: understanding the value and purpose of the agencies involved, the needs they must address, and the environment in which they operate;
- *planning*: identifying the gaps between what is needed and what is available, then deciding how these gaps will be addressed;
- *doing*: securing services and ensuring they are delivered as planned; and
- *reviewing*: monitoring the impact of services and ensuring future commissioning activities take review findings into account.

The danger is that these complex activities are, in practice, reduced to a competitive tendering activity, often framed by a rigid set of costed outputs and complex contract conditions. As seen in Chapter 2, local authorities were required to radically shift their role from direct provision to commissioning. In so doing, they stepped into an unfamiliar world, one that is normally found in commercial business, such as sourcing providers, negotiating contracts and monitoring arrangements. The research conducted in the 1990s by Wistow et al (1994, 1996) revealed what a culture shock this was at the time for local councillors, officers and front-line staff, who were more accustomed to a traditional 'welfare state' model. It might be expected that since that time, there would be greater familiarity with the task and less resistance to the principle but this is not necessarily the case.

Today, around a third of all public expenditure is outsourced via 'procurement' (Pritchard and Lasko-Skinner, 2019) even though the record of achievement is, at best, mixed. The most spectacular recent failure was the collapse of the outsourcing giant Carillion, which had managed services across education, the NHS, prison services and transport. Other outsourced public services that have run into difficulty include the probation service, the prison service, rail franchising, the forensic science service, Learn Direct, court translation services, housing for asylum seekers, welfare benefit assessment, free schools and academies, and the NHS. Overall, evidence of successful outsourcing is remarkably thin on the ground.

A report from the New Local Government Network (2018) identified five core problems with the outsourcing model:

- *Territorial: siloed working within and between sectors.* The inward focus of many partners can lead to a preoccupation with contract management and the offloading of risk.
- *Process-driven: unimaginative and bureaucratic approaches.* A culture that encourages prescriptive ways of working discourages creativity and focuses on the minimisation of risk in the awarding of contracts. The procurement mission is seen as technical rather than strategic.
- *Rigid: contracts that are too restrictive.* Contracts that are too rigid and prescriptive can prevent opportunities to adapt or change course.
- *Closed door: weak transparency and accountability.* A closed-door culture can exclude the public from scrutinising decisions. Commercial confidentiality is used as a justification for restricting the provision of information to the public.
- *Linear: a narrow and centralised approach that neglects the creation of long-term value within places and systems.* This can lead to a blinkered view of complex systems and the unique assets of specific places.

Local authority commissioning of adult social care

It might be thought that adult social care – with almost three decades experience of implementing the 'purchaser–provider split' behind it – would be an exemplar of effective commissioning but there is little evidence to suggest that this is the case. Too often, commissioning has been reduced to a hand-to-mouth process devoid of a wider purpose. The skills and capacity to commission, contract and monitor have all been diminished by years of austerity, while the hollowing out of the main commissioning body – local government – has inherently weakened activity. Indeed, there often seems to be no strategy to harness the outsourcing of public services to some strategic direction; rather, the end product is simply market diversification in itself, with an assumed expectation of greater 'cost-effectiveness' (Committee on Standards in Public Life, 2018).

Crude cost savings have long since appeared to be the hallmark of adult social care commissioning. In general, councils have annually set a price they were willing to pay for care and support, a figure that reflected the reduced amounts of funding they were receiving from central government. In 2016, it was reported that 20 per cent of the savings that had been made by councils were achieved in this way (Institute of Public Care, 2016). This has had parlous consequences for the care market, especially small providers operating on low margins. Moreover, many councils appeared to be making no attempt to understand the costs of the care provision they were commissioning, leading to a ruling in the High Court (the 2010 Pembrokeshire Judgment) that councils must have in place a proper process to come to a view on the costs they were prepared to meet.

Given the limited success of single organisation commissioning, it is unsurprising that ambitious attempts to 'jointly commission' with other agencies (in order to deliver more joined-up services) also have a poor record of proven success (Hudson, 2011b). One comprehensive review of 600 research studies about the impact of joint commissioning (446 in health and 149 in social care) concluded that the quality of the studies relating to the impact of joint commissioning was low and there could be little confidence in them (Social Science Research Unit, 2012).

The Care Act 2014 imposed a new 'market-shaping' role on local authorities. Section 5(1) states that each local authority 'must promote the efficient and effective operation of a market in services for meeting care and support needs', with a view to ensuring that prospective 'customers' have a variety of high-quality providers from which to choose and sufficient information to make an informed decision. An indication of how well local authorities are meeting their market-shaping obligations might be expected to be found in the content of the local 'market position statements' that they are obliged to produce.

Early evidence on the sophistication of these strategic statements has not been encouraging. A review of the care home market by the Competition and Markets Authority (2017) looked at 20 local market position statements and found that none of them even presented estimates of additional future capacity needed. A more in-depth study of six localities led by the University of Birmingham found that market position statements were recognised by interviewees as a potential channel to communicate the local authority's vision for social care. However, the interviewees believed that, in their current form, the documents did not facilitate this and did not supply the data required to support providers' service development. It was noted in particular that the data within the statements were often focused on demographic projections rather than developing a vision as to how a holistic care system can respond to possible future demands (Needham et al, 2020).

Even if market position statements demonstrated more ambition and purpose, there are limits on the extent to which local authorities can shape the behaviour of independent companies providing services on their behalf. Indeed, the main legislative powers held by local authorities in relation to the non-statutory sector are less about actively shaping the market and more about reactively trying to stave off market failure. Although local authorities have responsibility for somehow 'managing' the care market, this is problematic, especially where large providers operate across multiple boundaries (LaingBuisson, 2018a):

- it is unclear who has complete oversight of that provider's operations;
- managing the transfer or closure becomes increasingly difficult when there are thousands of residents and a large number of organisations involved;
- high market concentrations at a regional level are challenging for individual local authorities to oversee;
- investors can have a wide-ranging portfolio of diverse international business interests, of which care provision is marginal;
- many providers are carrying substantial debt structured in complex arrangements; and
- the care market has close and complex interactions with other markets, such as property and finance.

Given the 30-year existence of adult social care commissioning, remarkably little is known about those whose actually undertake the task – their principles, outlook, background and training, and how they handle day-to-day dilemmas. An interesting insight is the research by Davies et al (2020) into the commissioning of home care, which found commissioners reporting enormous variation in how their roles were set up within their organisations and what the role entailed. The researchers found it difficult to identify a common definition but identified three distinct (and not necessarily mutually exclusive) roles.

First, the *overseeing role* involved supporting providers, setting up and maintaining contracts, and ensuring care was available for the population within an authority. It was presented as a mediating role, with some respondents articulating a narrative of trying to pre-empt difficulties and proactively prevent business failure for providers. This sort of mediating role was closely associated with having an open dialogue with providers.

The second role identified was the *strategic role*, with strategic leadership explicitly described as setting a 'direction' of travel, with the implication that this changed and developed over time. However, commissioners rarely articulated the underpinning rationale for their strategy or the reasons for changing it. The most frequently cited strategic priority was an ambition to become more outcome focused, which depended on working more closely with providers and changing inflexible contracts. This is a challenging role, and one that conflicted with other factors, such as the professional culture within public and private organisations, a poor understanding of outcomes, and a reluctance to change practice and systems that used 'time and task'.

The third feature of the commissioners' role – the *network development role* – involved creating networks and working closely with other areas of the local authority and beyond to ensure the smooth delivery of care. In this case, respondents often outlined complicated organisational arrangements, where the commissioner was part of a complex network of commissioning, procurement, contracting and quality monitoring. Some were part of joint commissioning units across local authorities, though few jointly commissioned with health. An important network for some commissioners was with local providers, who were regarded as bringing an understanding of and connection to the community in terms of local knowledge and commitment:

> These different approaches are difficult balancing acts to undertake. Most interviewees were striving to improve the relationship with providers whilst also maintaining clear transactions in the form of contract specifications. However, commissioners reported tensions between contracting that involved detailed and prescriptive specifications, and collaborating with providers, acknowledging that care could not be regarded as a transactional process. (Davies et al, 2020)

Staffing continuity and capacity is a further problem here. Needham et al (2020) identify the problems created by changing personnel within local authority commissioning departments due to staff cuts. From the provider perspective, a key barrier to trust can be the high turnover of local authority commissioners, care managers and social workers, which inhibits communication, continuity and a coherent organisational long-term strategy. At the same time, it can negatively affect institutional memory within the local authority to the detriment of a coherent and planned approach to social care provision and market shaping.

In the meantime, commissioners are often beset by factors outside of their control. Cost is probably the most important of these but others also make it difficult to secure an effective outcome. Providers retain responsibility for the workforce and, more fundamentally, the business owners retained the right to exit the market if arrangements are not to their satisfaction. Local authorities have a duty under Section 5 of the Care Act 2014 to promote the efficient and effective operation of a market in care services, including an obligation to 'have regard for the importance of fostering a workforce whose members are able to ensure the delivery of high-quality services'. It is not clear how this obligation can be met, particularly in the case of services paid for by those who fund their own care.

Attempts to be more innovative in the commissioning process can easily be stymied. Within a local authority, attempts to shape the market do not just rest on those with direct responsibility for social care commissioning, but can also require the support of other departments, such as procurement and legal teams, as well as services such as housing and planning. Needham et al (2020: 30) found that 'several commissioners discussed how they had experimented with partnership approaches – including co-designing approaches with providers and other stakeholders – but had to abandon this approach due to internal resistance from legal and procurement teams and an inclination to emphasise contract price'. It is in such circumstances that Davies et al (2020) conclude that the relationship between the commissioner and the provider is poised in a delicate balance between vulnerability and power.

Commissioning from the third sector

If the relationship between local authorities and the private sector is often fraught, it might be thought that the relationship with long-standing partners in the third sector would be better. Again, however, the complexity of the sector creates a difficult relationship. The Charity Commission (2020) estimates that there are 167,000 voluntary and community sector organisations in England and Wales, most of them small and community-based, with 90 per cent operating on an annual income of less than £500,000. Of the 167,000, some 36,000 are thought to provide health and social care services. In an echo of the situation in the private sector, Baird et al (2018) report ongoing unhelpful commissioning practices by local authorities in terms of accessing and securing funding.

Commissioning agencies have strong imperatives to ensure continuity, consistency, equity and accountability, whereas third sector agencies are independent organisations that have developed their own cultures and ways of working (Institute for Local Governance, 2018). A front-line perspective from Newcastle Council for Voluntary Service (2018), for example, notes the tendency for commissioners and procurement officers within local authorities to work in separate teams. This can mean that those commissioners who have an interest in running new and more flexible procedures may be charged with having insufficient understanding of procurement constraints. The report also finds a tendency to bring together sets of smaller contracts into large single-tender opportunities that encourage larger bidders at the expense of smaller groupings. It is in these circumstances that the National Council for Voluntary Organisations (NCVO, 2019) reports that the bulk of grant income to the third sector goes to the largest charities with an annual income of £10 million or more, even though these larger charities make up only 0.43 per cent of the total voluntary sector.

These dilemmas have led some to conclude that procurement and contract management tools that are appropriate for buying highly commoditised and easily specified goods and services are not appropriate for commissioning complex support services and front-line human services. The shift from a relational form of contracting heavily based on personal relationships and institutional trust to a highly transactional approach is based upon a failure to understand this distinction (Sturgess, 2018). Failures in commissioning will obviously impact upon the appropriateness and effectiveness of support. In its annual review of performance, adult social care regulator the Care Quality Commission (2019) concluded that people too often had to chase around different care services to access even basic support, and that in the worst cases, they ended up in crisis or with the wrong kind of care.

The mixed record of local authority commissioning is, however, only part of the dilemma of commissioning in a market setting. Although local authorities were the dominant commissioners at the outset of the quasi-market model in the early 1990s, there has since been a growth in two other commissioning sources – those of direct payments (or variants of this model) and those who pay for all or some of their own care (self-funders). This has hugely complicated the situation by creating parallel commissioning activity at the macro and micro levels – a potential tension between standardisation and customisation (Needham, 2018).

The growth of direct payments

Direct payments in adult social care are sums of money allocated by a local authority to service users to be spent on services to meet their care needs. They can be managed on behalf of users by the authority or a third party, or given directly to users to spend themselves. Variants on this model have evolved over the last three decades. The passing of the Community Care (Direct Payments) Act 1996 meant that from 1 April 1997, local authorities were given the permissive power to make cash payments, or a mix of services and cash, in lieu of local authority-commissioned services to those disabled people who were willing and able to take responsibility for their own care arrangements. Initially, these payments were available only to people aged between 18 and 65 but eligibility was extended to those aged over 65 from February 2000, and then to carers, parents of disabled children, and 16 and 17 year olds from April 2001. In April 2003, regulations came into force that changed the *power* to offer direct payments to a *duty* to do so, thereby requiring councils to offer direct payments to all people using community care services.

As noted in Chapter 2, the idea of direct payments came in the first instance from the disability movement itself and was rooted in the belief that those using services should have greater choice and control over the support they bought (or commissioned) to meet their assessed care needs. In 2007, the government introduced the broader concept of a 'personal budget' – again, a sum of money allocated to an adult to meet their assessed social care needs. The Care Act 2014 went further and required local authorities to give all eligible users a personal budget from April 2015, thereby embedding this notion of 'personalised commissioning' into the legal framework for adult social care – and for the first time, those in residential settings were also included. Since 2014, the NHS has also been introducing personal budgets into healthcare (National Audit Office, 2016). An extension of the law in relation to personal health budgets in December 2019 meant that people using wheelchairs or needing mental health support under Section 117 of the Mental Health Act could also have access.

The number of people in receipt of personal budgets has increased from 65,000 in 2008 to around 500,000 by 2019 (Martinez and Pritchard, 2019) and the *NHS Long Term Plan* (NHS England, 2019b) envisages 200,000 people using a personal health budget by 2024. Although attractive in principle, this model is not without difficulty.

The first problem is market unresponsiveness. Fox (2018) notes that there has been little development of affordable, tailored new care services designed to help people stay active, social and connected; rather, a personal budget might simply mean choosing from a list of care providers offering a pared-down version of the traditional service that would previously have been purchased by the council. Second, the level of funding is low, limiting the scope of the budget to basic levels of personal care. Finally, there may be an unresponsive culture of 'standardisation' within local authorities, one that inhibits the creative use of personal budgets. Holders of budgets might be expected to undertake all of the administration and accounting procedures unaided, and then be monitored on how the budget is spent rather than upon how their lives within the community can be enhanced (Think Local Act Personal, 2018).

Although the personal budget model worked well for many disabled adults of working age, their application to older people has been more difficult. The main barriers to greater uptake have been identified as: poorly informed care managers; lack of direct payments support services; lack of enthusiasm among local authorities; poor public information; overly complicated monitoring systems; and difficulties with associated responsibilities (Davey et al, 2007). Carr (2013) reported that the majority of older people receiving personal budgets and direct payments were using them for personal care rather than to support social and community activities. She concluded that the present generation of older people may be different from the coming generations in terms of expectations, but for now, it appeared that people in later life were less likely to want to take on responsibility for managing their budget and organising their care and support.

This shift towards 'personalised commissioning' is consistent with the critique of the Seebohm state model of the 1970s and raises some important implications for policy and practice. Once again, the role of the social worker is diminished, both in terms of assessing and arranging care packages, and in terms of offering a direct professional service. More fundamentally, the model could be seen as the triumph of neoliberalism, with individuals purchasing their own care (albeit with public funding) and thereby transferring control from public sector agencies to individuals. Feelings run high: some see it as the incarnation of neoliberalism; those able to make use of the payments often feel a sense of control and empowerment; and many others view it as a model that is attractive in principle but flawed in implementation (West, 2013).

The rise of 'self-funders'

The widespread denial of access to local authority-funded support, a stringent means test that has remained unchanged for a decade and an explosion in housing equity has resulted in an unplanned growth in the number of people paying for their own care – 'self-funders'. People either completely funding their own care or making top-up payments are now estimated to be around 45 per cent of all users, much the same as for those entirely funded by local councils. Moreover, those in this position typically pay a 40 per cent premium for residential and nursing care compared with the usual rate paid by local authorities (Competition and Markets Authority, 2017). Any shift in the equilibrium between self-funders and council-funded users could have profound implications for social care providers. Should there be a significant increase in the proportion of those in receipt of council-funded support relative to self-funders (say, through a more generous means test), then some providers could find many of their self-funding users suddenly becoming eligible for council support and no longer cross-subsidising their operations. The chances of this happening seem to be high.

As noted earlier, there is a substantial gap between what is being charged by most care home providers and what the council is prepared to pay for via the commissioning process. This leaves those wishing to enter (or continue to stay in) a more expensive care home facing the problem of how to bridge the financial gap via 'top-ups'. These amounts are not small and would weigh heavily upon the resources of ordinary families. A detailed investigation by the Just Group (2019) calculated the average annual fee for self-funders to be £44,252 compared to a typical sum of £31,720 for council-funded residents. A total of 90 per cent of care homes were estimated to be operating this differential pricing policy in 2019, compared to around 20 per cent in 2005. This leaves a substantial gap for 'top-up' payments to meet from personal sources – an average of over £12,000 in England, with the highest in the South East (over £18,000) and the lowest in the North East (over £5,000). This is resulting in a growing polarisation of the market, with some providers turning exclusively to self-funders.

Future prospects for this source of funding look problematic. Fewer pensioners will get defined benefits pensions over the next decade, making it even harder for them to pay for their care. It is estimated that only around the top 10 per cent of retired households by income can afford to pay the fees charged by nursing homes (Irwin Mitchell, 2020). Although people of pensionable age could release an estimated

£1.2 trillion in equity by moving out of homes with two or more spare bedrooms, this requires heroic assumptions to be made about the alternative housing options that are available. It also goes against the grain of the political priority frequently given to the avoidance of selling homes to pay for care costs.

Given the huge numbers of people making a contribution towards their care costs, surprisingly little seems to be known about them. Henwood et al (2018) note that in the majority of local authorities, a proactive offer of support and care planning to self-funders would be seen as completely revolutionary. Indeed, there even seems to be little evidence that councils are engaged in forward planning for those transiting from self-funding to council funding as their resources are run down. Henwood et al point out that if people make poor financial planning choices and run out of money faster, they will fall back more quickly on local authority support, yet this might be the first time they become known to the council. It is estimated that about a quarter of self-funders do run out of money in this way – a significant financial risk for councils and a dereliction of their commissioning responsibility.

Even if more was known about the numbers of self-funders, this does little to strengthen their position as effective commissioners of their own care and support. A market requires 'customers' who seek and digest information to inform their choice of product. From this perspective, the care home market in particular has some characteristics of an inefficient market (National Audit Office, 2011): entry is often unplanned and made in response to a personal crisis; and there are very low rates of switching to a different provider in the event of dissatisfaction. Selecting care in this way is what economists conceptualise as an 'experience good' – one in which the exact nature of the service is not known until after purchase. The obstacles facing those who fund their own support has been comprehensively identified by the Competition and Markets Authority (2017), which notes that: most individuals and families are poorly informed and have done little or no planning or research; they struggle with the notion of exercising choice and rarely move between providers; there are low levels of complaints and fears of retaliation in the event of making one; and there is a lack of understanding of the formal complaints procedure.

Notwithstanding difficulties with both of these forms of 'personal commissioning', the market position of those who self-fund is often weaker than those receiving a personal budget from a local authority. Baxter et al (2019) note that the ideology of consumerism ran in parallel with economic arguments for markets and choice – the latter is portrayed as an intrinsic good, being the key to citizenship, autonomy and independence. An important assumption here is the availability and quality of information, and the capacity to use that information. A system of sorts has evolved to support holders of personal budgets but not self-funders, who often struggle to find and understand information about social care, and rarely consider approaching their local council for advice. They can end up disadvantaged and isolated, with care arrangements made by chance rather than active choice (Henwood and Hudson, 2008). Additionally, the post-purchase appropriateness of care that self-funders receive is not monitored in the same way as that of holders of personal budgets.

Commissioning and austerity

Regardless of the level and mode of commissioning, all activity will be to no avail without adequate resources to purchase provision. Toynbee and Walker (2020) refer to the period between 2010 and 2020 as 'the lost decade' – one that witnessed 'a drive to renew and harden anti-state and anti-tax individualism, testing them to destruction'. Over this time, core government funding to local councils is estimated to have fallen by around £15 billion – a near 60 per cent reduction in real terms. This is an unprecedented and quite astonishing statistic. Although adult social care is delivered and mainly funded locally, decisions by central government strongly shape how much money local authorities have to do this; in turn, this makes adult social care a national as well as a local responsibility.

Under the influence of a nationally imposed austerity policy, councils cut spending on adult social care by almost 10 per cent between 2009/10 and 2014/15. This reversed the trend in the early 2000s, when spending increased by an average of 5.7 per cent in real terms each year (Institute for Government, 2019). In turn, this has led to a tightening of eligibility criteria for the assessment of need and had huge implications for the availability of provision. The Local Government Association (2020c) estimates that adult social care faces an additional future funding requirement of around £2.6 billion for 2020/21 and almost £8 billion by 2024/25. Even in the unlikely event that these sums are met, it would only cover the 'provider market gap' (the difference between what providers say is the cost of delivering care and what councils currently pay) and 'core pressures', such as paying for the mandatory increases in the National Living Wage.

Moreover, these cuts bear more heavily on some parts of the country than others. Although the rules on entitlement to publicly funded adult social care are set nationally, access to social care varies depending on where people live. Unlike the NHS, each local authority makes its own decisions about budgets and services, so some spend more than others. Some of this variation may constitute a reasonable response to local circumstances but it can also reflect the different amounts of money local authorities get from government and from raising council tax. The authorities that can raise the least through council tax tend to be the most deprived areas, which, on average, have most need to spend on social care. This may affect the amount and quality of care providers available, not just for publicly funded care users, but for self-funders too (Bottery, 2019).

Burn and Needham (2020) note that 'austerity' is a catch-all term and go on to identify several distinct parameters:

- *Lack of access to services*: limited access to services is evident despite the explicit promises of the Care Act to improve support for users and carers. Falling capacity in the sector is also linked to low local authority fees, especially in relation to nursing homes.
- *Risk aversion and tighter local authority control*: although constrained resources might be seen as a driver for innovation, the greater likelihood is that austerity will lead to risk aversion and a compliance approach.
- *Short-termism*: short-term resource pressures to meet current demand conflict with the more long-term and relationship-building aspects required for prevention and market shaping.
- *Low trust between partners*: the financial difficulties faced by providers can affect the closeness of their relationship with the local authority, with providers taking a defensive stance to protect their business interests rather than engaging with attempts to shape the market. This lack of trust between commissioners and providers can make it very hard to build up long-term relationships that might enable the co-design of new models of support.
- *Fatalism*: to some extent, the impact of constrained resources can induce fatalism about the likelihood of receiving support, which, in turn, can depress demand. Negative national and local press coverage about the 'care crisis' can reduce people's sense of what is possible.

All of this takes its toll on users and carers in terms of unmet need. Age UK (2019) estimates that there are 1.5 million older people in England who need some help with day-to-day life but do not receive it. Many will have been 'signposted' to a diminishing voluntary sector; evidence on the effectiveness of this sort of response is not collected nationally or locally. Indeed, we know very little at all about the scale and consequences of unmet need. Data from the Malnutrition Task Force (2020) suggest that the number of older people diagnosed with malnutrition has more than trebled to almost 500,000 in the past decade, and that one in ten people over the age of 65 are malnourished or at risk of malnutrition. As the vast majority of people affected live at home, this often goes unnoticed. Again, the English Longitudinal Study of Ageing (Banks et al, 2019) found over 230,000 people aged 75+ having difficulty with the physicality of eating, such as cutting up food, and 1.9 million having difficulty eating because of a dental condition – simple matters to correct but that can have very harmful consequences when untended.

Even where access to support is secured, austerity can lead to an impersonal and inappropriate response. As noted by the Local Government Association (2020a), the tendency is to define a person by what they cannot do, then assess whether these needs are eligible for support. If they are, the person becomes a 'service user', whose needs are secondary to those of 'the system'. The report astutely observes that, 'In essence social care faces the frequently impossible task of having to distil the notion of a good life into a set of services that, in turn, are prioritised and rationed' (Local Government Association, 2020a: 4).

Informal carers will also bear the brunt of denial of access to formal support. Estimates from Carers UK (2019b), for example, suggest that half of women will undertake a caring role by the age of 46 (compared to men, who can expect to do so by 57). Of those doing so for more than 50 hours a week, almost half report that their finances had been negatively impacted, 52 per cent had suffered poorer physical health and 77 per cent were suffering from stress or anxiety. There are now reckoned to be 8.8 million people in the UK providing informal care to a family member or friend – more than ever before – and over a third of them spend well over half of their time (day and night) caring for a family member or friend (NHS Digital, 2019a). Moreover, these are not short-term commitments: nearly a third had been caring for 15 years or more and 15 per cent for ten to 14 years. At the same time, the increasing burden on unpaid carers threatens to undo some of the progress made in raising female employment rates over the past 20 years, particularly among older women. The Care Act 2014 stipulates the duty of local authorities to assess carers' needs for support but the *State of Caring Survey* by Carers UK (2019a) found that only 27 per cent of the 7,525 participating carers had been assessed or offered an assessment in the previous 12 months.

Chapter summary

This chapter has focused upon the ways in which 'commissioning' has been developed and applied at the organisational and individual levels. In broad terms, 'commissioning' refers to the process of planning and the strategic purchasing of services. It might be thought that adult social care – with almost three decades of experience of implementing the 'purchaser–provider split' behind it – would be an exemplar of effective commissioning but there is little evidence to suggest that this is the case. Too often, commissioning has been reduced to a hand-to-mouth process devoid of a wider purpose.

Relatively little is known about those whose task it is to actually commission adult social care but research suggests that there is enormous variation in how the roles are set up and what they entail. From the provider perspective, a key barrier to trust can be the high turnover of local authority commissioners, care managers and social workers, which inhibits communication, continuity and a coherent organisational long-term strategy. In the case of commissioning from the voluntary sector, there is evidence of unhelpful commissioning practices by local authorities in terms of accessing and securing funds.

Failures in commissioning also impact upon the appropriateness and effectiveness of support, and the emergence of direct payments/ personal budgets – sums of money allocated by a local authority to service users to be spent on services to meet their care needs. Although the personal budget model worked well for many disabled adults of working age, their application to older people has been more difficult. The widespread denial of access to local authority-funded support, along with a stringent means test that has remained unchanged for a decade, has resulted in an unplanned growth in the number of people paying for their own care – 'self-funders' – about whom surprisingly little seems to be known.

Between 2010 and 2020, core government funding to local councils is estimated to have fallen by around £15 billion – a near 60 per cent reduction in real terms. All of this takes its toll on users and carers in terms of unmet need. It is estimated that there are 1.5 million older people in England who need some help with day-to-day life but do not receive it. Even where access to support is secured, austerity can lead to an impersonal and inappropriate response. Informal carers will also bear the brunt of denial of access to formal support.

4

Dilemmas in the provision of adult social care

Introduction

Chapter 2 charted the emergence and consolidation of the privatisation of provision of adult social care in England. This has resulted in significant investment by private businesses, especially in residential and nursing care. The precise amounts are difficult to estimate but some within the sector put it at around £30 billion and rising (LaingBuisson, 2014). This is a significant amount and if the money saved by the Treasury had gone into other ways of boosting adult social care, there would be no talk of it being 'in crisis'. In considering some of the problems thrown up by the privatisation of provision, it is therefore important not to undervalue the scale of this investment. Those hoping for a rapid and substantial 'renationalisation' of the sector would certainly have to make a calculation of the sums expended and the costs of compensation that would be required. Chapter 5 examines this issue further.

Nevertheless, this situation has also created problems that would probably have been less likely to occur with a state-run model. Four such concerns will be examined in this chapter: availability; fragility; exploitation and profiteering; and workforce issues.

Availability

Chapter 3 questioned whether the services and support commissioned are well suited to meeting individual needs and preferences, and examined the declining resource base available for the purchase of provision. However, since private businesses will only operate where the financial rewards are deemed acceptable, there are liable to be problems relating to the availability of *any* form of care in some places. Evidence suggests that care home places are disappearing from areas that already have a shortfall of beds, while new high-quality facilities are opening for those who can pay their own way – a distinct two-tier system in every respect (CSI Market Intelligence, 2020). Indeed, a CSI Market

Intelligence (2020) report notes that of the 20 local authorities that gained most beds, ten were already oversupplied, and at the other end of the scale, 12 out of the 20 local authorities that lost the most beds were already undersupplied.

Even if local authority funding was improved, a pattern of provision dependent upon the investment decisions of a multiplicity of autonomous businesses will not necessarily respond to the scale and distribution of need. Private companies will set up and deliver services where business opportunities seem most attractive, and will close them where the return on investment is perceived as inadequate. Moreover, there is no strategic planning apparatus that has the authority, power and remit to ensure the availability of provision. This can result in a geographical lottery of service availability in which some areas of the country have become 'care deserts', even for those who self-fund. Sometimes, this is because there are no providers; on other occasions, it is because although there are providers, they have insufficient numbers of staff.

Research into these 'care deserts' (Incisive Health, 2019) has focused on four key market indicators: the availability of a workforce; care home beds; care home beds with nursing; and the domiciliary care market. For each of these, evidence was found to suggest that the adult social care market is not operating in a way capable of providing care to everyone who needs it:

- The social care workforce crisis is worsening, with vacancy rates rising. In some areas of the country, the lack of specialist workers in particular is now severely limiting the care that providers are able to offer.
- The number of care home beds has reduced over the last five years at a time of rising need. These reductions are not evenly distributed around the country, leaving provision in some areas even more precarious.
- The situation for care home beds with nursing is even more acute. Despite a slight rise in the total number of beds nationally over the last five years, some local areas have lost more than a third of their nursing beds over the last three years.
- The domiciliary care market is in crisis, with the number of hours of care provided falling by three million over the last three years.

This situation contrasts sharply with the pre-market era of the 1960s and 1970s, when local authorities were assumed to hold responsibility for ensuring that services were available to meet eligible need – and, indeed, were tasked by central government with producing plans to do so. In 1962, and again in 1972, local authorities were required to prepare ten-year plans for community social services (Wistow, 2012). The fact that both turned out to be largely paper exercises (the last in particular was based on unrealistic guidelines about available resources) does not detract from the significance of the exercises. Again, in 1977, social services departments were asked by the Department of Health and Social Security (DHSS) to submit a written account of their future strategies and priorities, along with statements of their expected expenditure, capital and current, broken down by client group for the following three years, together with population and provision figures for each client group. In this case, 'norms' were recommended by the DHSS for separate client groups, typically workers or places per thousand population (Glennerster, 1981).

This sort of oversight and planning – for all of its faults – no longer exists in adult social care, though it continues to be an expectation in respect of hospitals and schools. This contrast might say something about the difference in respective value that is placed upon these three services, with the scale and distribution of adult social care provision seemingly of little interest to the state. There is still a concern about how to achieve a better balance between greater standardisation of care provision at the national level and allowing flexibility to respond to local needs. The Care Act 2014 does set out national eligibility criteria for care and support but there is a great deal of local discretion – councils may meet their obligations by whatever means they choose provided they can justify that this meets the needs of their local population and of individuals who qualify for support.

The capricious nature of availability on the part of the private sector is mirrored by that of the voluntary and community sector. Research for the think tank New Philanthropy Capital (Corry, 2020) demonstrates that charitable wealth and resources – from volunteers to philanthropic donations and council grants – is disproportionately concentrated in England's most affluent areas at the expense of the country's least affluent communities. Deprived areas in general suffer from a lack of charities, compounding economic hardship with a lack of organised social capital. The report argues that this is not an accident; rather, it is influenced by the charity taxation regime and the way that independent funders and larger charities behave. It calls for a rebalancing of public funding and philanthropy to rebuild civil society – broadly defined as local charities, clubs and community and voluntary groups – in the 'left behind' areas of the North and Midlands.

Fragility

A related dilemma to service availability is that of market fragility – businesses move into the market and they move out. The most serious problem with the creation of a market in social care is the prospect of significant market failure, and the impact of this on people who are at very vulnerable points in their lives. This is not so much a question of small individual providers failing to meet regulatory standards and being deregistered; rather, it is the prospect of one or more major providers covering thousands of service users exiting the care market, or of multiple smaller providers doing the same.

During the 1980s and 1990s, care home closures were not uncommon as the market began to adapt to the introduction of new regulatory standards, and it became common for consolidations within the industry to take place. Smaller operators were increasingly bought out by larger operators or were simply closed because they could not generate sufficient economies of scale to survive. As larger operators began to hold more influence in the sector, the state became increasingly reliant on a smaller number of larger-scale private providers, often backed by private equity companies. The potential for a large-scale market failure then became a distinct possibility, especially in the wake of the global economic crisis of 2008 and the decision by the Westminster government in England to prioritise reductions in local government spending (and hence on social care) as a prime austerity measure.

In 2011, the first major casualty was Southern Cross – a large national care home provider that had 9 per cent of the market nationally but a much greater share in certain regional areas. Not the least of the problems here was the remote ownership of the company – a complex mix of creditors, property investors, bondholders, banks, shareholders and landlords. The collapse of Southern Cross was the first major occasion when the interests of private companies had come face to face with the need for service continuity for highly vulnerable people. It also brought the market model into public discourse in a new and politically explosive manner (Scourfield, 2012) as councils sought to protect residents, and central government began to take the problem of market failure seriously.

A review of the stability of the care market in England at the time (Institute of Public Care, 2014) identified a range of reasons for the collapse of Southern Cross: a rental bill of £250 million per annum following the sale and leaseback of its properties; a drop in income that resulted in a reduction in property maintenance, which, in turn, led to lower occupancy; loans attracting higher interest rates because the company no longer had properties against which to secure loans; a fall in market confidence and share price; and poor management and quality of care, which led to adverse inspection reports and further decreases in occupancy levels. In effect, Southern Cross was in a downward market spiral with no way of ensuring continuity of care.

Much of the Southern Cross provision was eventually taken over by another major provider, Four Seasons, which has since befallen precisely the same fate as Southern Cross. The 'Big Four' care home groups (accounting for 14 per cent of all beds) were all up for sale in 2020. Three of them (HC–One, Barchester and Care UK) had been for sale for over a year and the other (Four Seasons) had been placed into administration (House of Commons Library, 2019a). Four Seasons, owned by a complex private equity fund, has been attempting to refinance its £565 million debt for over two years. In October 2019, it failed to pay the £10 million monthly rent on its 320 homes, which housed 16,000 residents and employed 22,000 care workers. Currently, it is in the hands of a Connecticut-based hedge fund (H/2 Capital Partners), having changed hands four times in 13 years among private equity firms. Over 80 per cent of Four Seasons residents are funded by local authorities, and if or when these homes are closed or sold, councils have a duty to find places for them. It is far from clear how this can be achieved.

This fragility is not confined to large companies. The Association of Directors of Adult Social Services (ADASS, 2018) reported providers ceasing to trade across home and residential care in more than a hundred council areas in only six months of 2018/19, as well as providers handing back contracts to more than 60 councils. This is consistent with more recent figures indicating that 45 per cent of providers have handed back contracts to local authorities, with 52 per cent also saying that they would need to do so in the near future (HFT, 2020). Similarly, in its annual review of the sector, the King's Fund (Bottery and Babalola, 2020) notes the problem of ongoing fragility amid reports of companies continuing to hand back contracts or go out of business. It is in such circumstances that the care regulator felt impelled to describe the market model as being at a 'tipping point' (Care Quality Commission, 2017b).

Exploitation and profiteering

Most of the adult social care sector consists of small for-profit companies operating on small margins and not-for-profit companies, again typically small and local in nature. However, as noted earlier, large profit-maximising companies have made significant incursions into the sector. It is here, and notably in relation to care homes, that accusations of exploitation and profiteering are particularly relevant (Care Quality Commission, 2020).

The most comprehensive attempt to follow the flow of money received by private companies running care homes is that by the CHPI (2019), which examined the accounts of 830 adult care home companies, and especially the 26 largest providers. Collectively, these companies represented 68 per cent of the total estimated revenue for independent adult social care home providers. The report identifies a number of forms of what it terms 'leakage', that is, money that is diverted away from direct care for residents, much of it in an opaque manner:

- *property costs:* rent for using the care home that is paid to an external company or a company with the same ownership as the care home;
- *debt repayments:* payments to banks, bondholders or other investors (at high interest rates), often to pay back a loan used to buy the company in the first place;
- *directors' remuneration:* payments for managing the business and its finances;
- *management fees:* costs charged to the company by a parent company for managing its finances and business functions;
- *offshore ownership:* this allows tax to be avoided when money is paid to related companies that are based overseas;
- *splitting up the company:* care home businesses are often split into multiple companies with the care home branch charged rent and management fees by the other companies, making the business look less profitable than it is; and
- *sale and leaseback:* many of the large companies sell their care home properties to a buyer then agree to rent them back for a high-cost rent.

In the case of the biggest 26 companies (accounting for 30 per cent of the market), the report calculated an average 'leakage rate' of 10 per cent, equivalent to a total of £1.5 billion. The rates are higher for private-equity-style ownership (13.35 per cent) than for small to medium-sized companies (7 per cent). The findings of a similar investigation by the Competition and Markets Authority (2017) were even more alarming, estimating that £20 out of every £100 put in goes to profit before tax, rent payments, management fees and interest are paid out.

Despite its high debts and market vulnerability, Four Seasons still awarded £2.4 million over two years to its highest-paid director and over £10 million to all of its directors. In 2019, HC-One, the largest care home provider, paid out £6 million to shareholders in dividends and an £800,000+ pay package to its highest-paid executive – double what was paid the previous year. Barchester, another large company, awarded its highest-paid director £915,000 in 2019, a rise of £230,000 over two years. While these handsome sums are being distributed, payment of tax is minimised by the use of tax havens. The parent companies of HC-One and Barchester are based in Jersey, while Four Seasons has selected Guernsey (Birrell, 2020).

There is a huge irony in these companies demanding that the state should increase fee levels when they take such steps to avoid making their own contribution to the state's finances. Residential adult social care is a low-risk activity since demand does not fall or vary, and taxpayers cover most of the cost on half of all beds; it is a stable market on which low returns on investment should be expected. The leakages identified in the CHPI and Competition and Markets Authority investigations leave these large private operators with returns on investment in excess of 12 per cent – margins that would normally only be expected in the most risky of markets (Centre for Research on Socio-Cultural Change, 2016).

It is reasonable to assume that the market share of these 'chain' companies will continue to increase, especially in residential care, where they have the major advantage of easy access to capital that they can use to update old homes and build new ones. The interest is strongest in that part of the market for those funding their own care. One recent industry report on investment performance reported that 'Institutional interest is particularly strong at the prime end of the care home market with bidders willing to pay a premium for well-located, purpose-built homes positioned for the private pay market' (Knight Frank, 2020: 4). This trend is also evident in children's social care services, where financial engineering techniques have resulted in increased levels of debt and risk, alongside hugely hiked profits. One recent study of 16 of the largest provider organisations reported a return on investment of 17.4 per cent, a staggeringly high return for what is essentially a stable and low-risk market (Rome, 2020).

Effects on the workforce

In 2018, the adult social care workforce was estimated at around 1.62 million full-time-equivalent jobs and the number working in the sector at around 1.49 million (Skills for Care, 2018c). These figures exclude an estimated 145,000 personal assistants employed by those arranging their own care and support (National Audit Office, 2018c). The sector is also growing, with an increase of 21 per cent (275,000 jobs) since 2009, and females make up 82 per cent of the workforce. It is also an ageing workforce. Between 2010 and 2018, the proportion of employees in the sector aged 50 and over increased from 32.8 per cent to 39.5 per cent. Over the same period, the proportion of the workforce aged 16 to 29 fell from 20 per cent to 17.1 per cent (Skills for Care, 2018a).

The privatisation of provision has resulted in a multiplicity of independent providers acting as autonomous businesses, each holding responsibility for employing, training and setting the pay, terms and conditions for their own workforce. Since the biggest single cost of providing personal care – around 60 per cent – is the front-line staff who deliver it, this is also the area where for-profit providers are likely to make operational returns in order to sustain profit margins. This is especially the case over the past decade, when public spending reductions have tightened operating margins. All of this has resulted in some specific problems for direct care staff, many of them reflecting the way in which the wider workforce has been restructured in the 'gig economy' (McBride and Smith, 2018). The employment situation of those providing front-line care has three defining features: low pay, insecurity and low status.

Low pay

A review back in 2014 by the House of Commons Public Accounts Committee (2014) reported evidence that: care workers' median pay was as low as £7.90 per hour; those working in community settings were frequently not paid for travelling time; and up to 220,000 direct care workers were being paid below the statutory minimum wage. Subsequent analysis by the Institute for Public Policy Research (IPPR, 2018b) has further revealed that adult social care accounts for a significant proportion of all low-paid workers in the UK. In 2018, 517,000 jobs in social care were paying below the real living wage, amounting to nearly one in ten of all jobs paying below this level. Given the gendered nature of the workforce, this also constitutes a significant factor behind the male–female pay gap.

Employers will also look to hold down the overall pay bill in other ways, notably, by flattening rewards for career progression – the pay differential between care workers with less than one year of experience and those with over 20 years has reduced to just 0.15p per hour. In turn, this raises the prospect of competition from other prospective employers, with the average hourly pay in adult social care typically below the basic rate paid in supermarkets.

Insecurity

Workplace insecurity arises most explicitly from the use of zero-hours contracts, whereby employees have no guarantee of how much work they might have and when they would be required to attend, receive no sick pay or holiday pay, and have no entitlement to employer pension schemes. According to data collected by Skills for Care (2018a), one in four workers in adult social care in England were on a zero-hours contract, rising to over half in the case of those in the domiciliary care sector. On top of this, there may be 'hidden' internal practices, such as restricting annual leave, reducing the numbers of qualified nursing staff, increasing resident–staff ratios, moving to unpaid online training to be completed at home, removing paid breaks and failing to pay for handover meetings at the start and end of shifts (Burns et al, 2016).

Low status

In addition to low pay and insecurity, the low status of care work is reflected in other ways: lack of regulation; low levels of education and training; weak career development; and gendered employment. The regulatory position of care workers in England is in stark contrast to other parts of the health and social work professions. While nurses, social workers, occupational therapists and others are regulated professions with mandatory training requirements, care workers in England have no professional regulation and no mandatory training. The regulatory issue remains unaddressed, but in the case of training, the Cavendish Review (2013) recommended common training standards across the health and social care sector through a Certificate of Fundamental Care. However, this qualification is not mandatory or enforced by a regulator, and concerns have been raised about quality assurance, portability and suitability (Allan et al, 2014). Take-up has accordingly been slow, with only a third having finished the course, which is intended to be completed within a short 12-week on-the-job period (Skills for Care, 2018a).

In turn, this means that opportunities for career progression are extremely limited. Rather than climb a career ladder, care workers stuck in a flat pay structure can easily be tempted away to other care services employers for small hourly increases in pay, resulting in a high volume of staff turnover. Alternatively, they will be tempted to find equally low-paid – but less demanding – work in other sectors of the economy. The deeply gendered nature of the workforce is a further factor here – females outnumber males by four to one and this feeds into the narrative that women are somehow expected to step in and provide care at low cost (Political Studies Association, 2016).

Although all sectors – statutory, private and voluntary – share the problems described earlier, there is nevertheless variation between them. Public sector and voluntary sector provision is now relatively marginal but, where available, it makes a difference across three dimensions – pay, security and education level:

- *Pay*: pay tends to be far lower in the private sector. Median hourly pay for the dwindling numbers of care workers still directly employed in the public sector in England in 2017 was £9.80, compared to just £7.76 for those employed by independent providers (Skills for Care, 2018a).
- *Security*: care workers employed by private companies in England are over three times more likely to be on zero-hours contracts than those employed in the public sector – 34.8 per cent compared to 10.1 per cent (Skills for Care, 2018a).
- *Education level*: over half (55.7 per cent) of care workers in the independent sector have no relevant social care qualifications, compared to just one in five (19.6 per cent) in the public sector (Skills for Care, 2018a). This is a situation that also seems to apply more widely across European Union (EU) countries (Eurofound, 2017).

These features of the workforce have developed, in part, because of the weakness of two potential countervailing variables: unionisation and workforce planning. In a largely privatised sector consisting of over 20,000 companies, the workforce has become atomised and lacking in bargaining power. Analysis of data by the IPPR (2018b) suggests that only one in five care workers (19.8 per cent) and senior care workers (20.6 per cent) are a member of a trade union or a staff association. In addition, the independent sector has very low levels of collective bargaining coverage. This leaves pay to be set by employers alone at a level dictated by the market – a sharp contrast to healthcare staff in the NHS, where pay and terms and conditions are collectively agreed nationally. Such nationally agreed terms and conditions were also the norm in adult social care prior to the creation of the market model, but as national and local government withdrew from actual service provision, so they also withdrew from their wage negotiation role with the workforce (Fair Work Convention, 2019). This situation has several deleterious effects: it discourages NHS staff from working in social care; it makes integrated working across the two sectors more difficult (House of Commons Public Accounts Committee, 2018); and it creates a gravitational pull among care workers towards a career in the NHS as a healthcare assistant (King's Fund et al, 2019).

At the national level, the Department of Health and Social Care is responsible for overseeing adult social care workforce planning in England; however, it has signally failed to undertake the task. A report by the National Audit Office (2018c) expressed astonishment at the absence of a national workforce strategy, noting that the last such strategy had been published a decade ago and was only available on a national archive web site. The Department of Health and Social Care funds and works in partnership with Skills for Care, a charity that aims to create a well-led, skilled and valued social care workforce. In 2017, this funding amounted to only £20 million, as compared to the £5 billion allocated to Health Education England, the body that leads on workforce planning in the NHS. At the local level, guidance issued under the Care Act 2014 states that public sector local authorities should encourage the training and development of care staff; however, these authorities have no powers to require providers to comply with any such demands.

It is also important to note that the split between the purchasing and provision of adult social care has had profound consequences for the long-standing profession of social work, which is now more focused on assessment and care planning rather than direct interventions. In the process, the education and training of social workers has itself become increasingly privatised, with traditional full-time university-based degrees in social work increasingly under threat from the government-funded 'fast-track' Frontline programme. Rather than the traditional model of full-time study interspersed with practice placements, Frontline consists of a five-week residential input, 12 months of on-the-job training and education, followed by a second year spent as a newly qualified social worker who is then considered to be qualified and ready to practice.

The programme has attracted controversy among academics for the limited understanding that can be acquired of the social science, psychosocial and sociolegal foundations of social work knowledge (Thoburn, 2017); however, the favourable government funding regime for fast-tracking compared with traditional courses is continuing to damage university undergraduate and postgraduate programmes (Skills for Care, 2018b). Indeed, for Tunstill (2019), this has amounted to an assault on all of the key mechanisms that have previously delivered a professionally qualified social worker, from qualifying to post-qualifying and continuing registration. In her view, this has substantially reduced the likelihood of social workers being able to take a socially critical position in their day-to-day work – a far cry from the 'radical social work' ethos of the pre-market era examined in Chapter 2.

Quality of care

Workforce issues

Eventually, all of these factors coalesce in a way that is harmful for those who have to rely upon services and support. The most notable impacts have been the failure to recruit sufficient staff and then to retain those that are recruited. The adult social care sector is simply an insufficiently attractive occupation, and without adequate staffing, there can be no adequacy of support.

There are an estimated 110,000 unfilled social care vacancies across the sector – a rate of 6.6 per cent compared with an average of 2.5 per cent across the economy in 2019. Although this is primarily a shortage of direct care staff, there are also problems with two other important staff categories. First, there is the registered manager role. Since 2010, the Care Quality Commission has required all regulated social care establishments to have a registered manager who is legally accountable for compliance with laws and regulations. In 2016/17, the vacancy rate for this category was 11.3 per cent, the highest across all care roles, with the National Audit Office (2018c) noting a discrepancy between the level of responsibility and the level of pay.

Second, there are registered nurses, of whom there must be at least one for each nursing home. Nursing staff are often paid less in a social care setting than if they worked in a healthcare setting. This has led many residential homes to withdraw nursing home beds and concentrate on providing only social care, despite the growing numbers of people with multiple and complex problems in need of nursing care (Department of Health, 2016). This has effects elsewhere within the NHS. Spiers et al (2019), for example, report that older adults' use of care homes may moderate hospital inpatient admissions and that, in particular, the presence of registered nurses in care homes may reduce the need to transfer residents to hospital.

In the meantime, it has been estimated that an extra 650,000 jobs will be needed by 2035 if the sector continues to grow at the current rate (Skills for Care, 2018a). This prospect is now further complicated by UK immigration policies and the departure of the UK from the EU. The social care sector has become increasingly reliant on migrant workers in recent years, with the number of workers joining the sector from the EU growing rapidly. There are around 95,000 EU nationals working in the social care sector, representing 7.8 per cent of care workers, and alongside them are 127,000 non-EU migrants, accounting for 9.5 per cent of the workforce (IPPR, 2018b). The Migration Advisory Committee (2018) set out recommendations to the government on a post-Brexit migration system that included a requirement that all skilled workers from outside the UK who have been living in the country for less than ten years will need to earn at least £30,000 a year to be allowed to settle permanently.

Some jobs, such as nursing, are exempt from this requirement; social care is not. The IPPR (2018b) estimates that 79 per cent of European Economic Area employees working full-time in social care would be ineligible to work in the UK under the skills and salary thresholds proposed by the Migration Advisory Committee. The subsequent Immigration (EU Withdrawal) Bill (Home Office, 2020) proposed a reduction in the earnings threshold to £25,600, with no adjustment for regional variations or differences across the UK. Given that the average salary in adult social care is estimated at just over £16,000, this will create huge recruitment problems for the sector. The government's view is that employers will need to adjust but it is not easy to see how this can be achieved when the sector is so starved of public funding.

The difficulties in recruiting staff are matched by problems in retaining them once they are in post. Industry staff turnover rates are alarmingly high (averaging around 30 per cent in 2017/18), leading providers to increasingly rely on expensive agency staff. Turnover is even higher for new care workers, nearly half (48 per cent) of whom leave within a year (House of Commons Communities and Local Government Committee, 2017). Recent figures from Skills for Care (2019) reveal: a turnover rate among those aged under 20 of 43.7 per cent; people leave soon after joining – turnover rates were 38.2 per cent for those with less than one year of experience in role; workers were more likely to leave if they were employed on zero-hours contracts (31.8 per cent turnover rate) compared to if they were not (24.9 per cent); and those paid more were less likely to leave their role.

Taken together, all of these trends can be predicted to have an adverse impact on the quality of care. If suitable staff cannot be recruited in the first place, there can be no adequacy of support; however, high staff turnover is also damaging. High-quality care also requires time for staff to build relationships with those they support and to have access to personalised support for their own continuing professional development. Too often, these are unavailable. When companies are fending off financial problems, the quality of the care that they provide has been found to diminish. In the case of care homes, the facilities deteriorate, staffing levels are reduced and additional 'services' for residents, such as outings or entertainment, are cut back (Benbow, 2008).

With domiciliary care, there has been wholesale adoption of a flawed 'task and time' model, with units of as little as 15 minutes per client imposed in order to reduce costs. One recent survey of home care workers (Unison, 2017b) reported insufficient time to prepare a meal (35 per cent), help with washing and bathing (30 per cent), toileting (30 per cent), or other personal matters such as stoma care (29 per cent). However, with excessive time pressure, it is the social aspect of care that is most commonly lost: 89 per cent felt that they did not even have time to chat.

Those working in adult social care are – or certainly should be – active moral agents, guided by ethical principles and making a critical interpretation of relevant ethical codes. However, as Julia Unwin (2018) notes, kindness, emotion and human relationships can too easily become the 'blind spot' in public policy. writing in the healthcare context Mannion (2014) goes even further, suggesting that there is an emerging consensus that caring and compassion are under threat – he refers to the 'compassion fatigue' associated with caring jobs that entail significant stress and investments of emotional labour.

Although care staff are widely – and rightly – seen as undertaking a demanding job very well in difficult circumstances, there have been widely reported accounts of grossly abusive and even criminal behaviour. The latter has most notably been in private healthcare facilities for adults with complex needs. Much of the abuse is low-level and related to stressful aspects of the work situation rather than the loss of an ethical compass. Cooper et al (2018), for example, conducted a large care home survey on the prevalence of abusive behaviour towards care home residents as reported by staff themselves over a three-month period. Some 'abuse' was reported in 91 out of 92 establishments, with neglect cited as the most common feature. This encompassed things like never being taken out of the home for enjoyment (34 per cent), no activity planned around a resident's interests (18 per cent), waiting for care (26 per cent), avoiding challenging behaviour (25 per cent), insufficient time with food (19 per cent) and insufficient care with moving (11 per cent). The authors note that staff are often caring for residents who resist care or are verbally or physically aggressive, and that they have little training and support to help them cope with these encounters.

It is not straightforward to put all of these variations down to sectoral provision. Although there are various data sets about social care provision, there are few accessible measures of quality with which to assess differences across the public, voluntary and private sectors. This is particularly the case with those who fund their own care. Nevertheless, an analysis by researchers at Future Care Capital (2019) teased out the following key findings:

- there are relatively few measures of quality that are publicly available with which to assess social care provision;
- Care Quality Commission inspection coverage and ratings have improved over time but are a lagging indicator of quality;
- the private sector tends to be rated as lower in quality than its public and not-for-profit counterparts;
- smaller care homes tend to be rated as better in quality than their larger counterparts; and
- social care-related quality of life is not obviously correlated to private company market share, but one reason for this may be that people who fully self-fund their care are excluded from the data sets.

Chapter summary

The privatisation of provision of adult social care in England has resulted in significant investment by private businesses in the sector, especially in residential and nursing care, and this has reduced the pressure on the Treasury to boost public sector investment. However, this situation has also created problems that would have been less likely to occur with a state-run model: availability; fragility; exploitation and profiteering; and effects on the workforce.

Private businesses will only operate where the financial rewards are deemed acceptable, so there are liable to be problems relating to the availability of *any* form of care in some places. A related dilemma to service availability is that of market fragility – businesses move into the market and they move out. The most serious problem with the creation of a market in social care is the prospect of significant market failure and the impact of this on people who are at very vulnerable points in their lives. The privatisation of provision has resulted in a multiplicity of independent providers acting as autonomous businesses, each holding responsibility for employing, training and setting the pay, terms and conditions for their own workforce.

Eventually, all of these factors coalesce in a way that is harmful for those who have to rely upon services and support. It is not straightforward to associate any particular quality of care with any specific sector, but there is evidence to suggest that the quality is higher in public and not-for-profit companies than in the private sector. This has fed into a long-running debate regarding the roles of the state and the market in adult social care, which is the topic of Chapter 5.

5

State or market?

Introduction

There are clearly problems with the operation of a market in adult social care; what is less evident is how to respond to this situation. Logically, there are three options: retain and reform the market; replace the market with a state-run service along the lines of the 1970s' model; and develop a new approach that is distinct from both of these options. This chapter is concerned with the first two options – put simply, state or market? Chapter 7 explores the scope for a third approach.

Renationalising the adult social care sector

As noted in Chapter 2, the outsourcing of public services to non-statutory providers, especially the private sector, has been the delivery model of choice in the UK for around 30 years. The budget devoted to such contracts is hard to estimate but is reckoned to be in excess of £100 billion (Walker and Tizard, 2018), equivalent to about 8 per cent of gross domestic product. The model has also changed in nature over the years, moving beyond back-office functions and into front-line service delivery.

A number of high-profile problems and outright failures have brought the limitations of this model into more prominent view. Perhaps the most spectacular was the collapse of the outsourcing giant Carillion, which managed services across education, the NHS, prison services and transport – indeed, 60 per cent of its work came from government contracts to deliver public services and facilities. The scathing inquiry by two joint committees of the House of Commons (House of Commons Business, Energy and Industrial Strategy Committee and Work and Pensions Committee, 2018) discovered not just incompetence, but ethical failings rooted in fecklessness, hubris and greed.

Concerns have also been raised across a number of other outsourced public services, including probation (HM Inspectorate of Probation, 2017; National Audit Office, 2019), the prison service (Dockley and Loader, 2016), the forensic science service (Commons Science and Technology Committee, 2016), the NHS (NHS Support Federation, 2017) and children's social care services (Jones, 2018). It is little wonder that in its inquiry into the wider issue of outsourcing and contracting, the Commons Public Administration and Constitutional Affairs Committee (2018) concluded that: it was unclear how and why the government decided whether to outsource a particular service; the evidence used to support outsourcing decisions was 'thin or non-existent'; and there had been a depressing inability to learn from repeated mistakes.

All of this has fuelled the popularity of calls to bring public services, the railways and the water and energy companies back under public control. This does not necessarily mean a return to top-down state control. The campaigning organisation We Own It (2019), for example, proposes the creation of a new democratically accountable organisation that would represent users and citizens, with publicly owned organisations run by a professional management team and governed by a supervisory board representing the public interest. This is all in line with the case put forward by Cumbers and Hanna (2019) for a new and more democratic approach – to develop forms of organisation and governance that stimulate public participation, increase accountability and empower communities and individuals that have traditionally been excluded.

Questions of implementation still remain, especially over how much the state would pay for requisitioned assets and how it would deal with potential legal challenges if the price was less than the market value. In the case of the failed bank Northern Rock, for example, the level of compensation was decided by Parliament but this transaction was relatively straightforward since the company assets were deemed worthless (House of Commons Committee of Public Accounts, 2016).

In the case of adult social care, the industry estimate is that investment has amounted to well over £30 billion and rising (LaingBuisson, 2014), and difficult decisions would have to be made on a number of aspects of renationalisation, such as:

- Would it apply to all non-statutory providers, private and not-for-profit alike?
- Would it apply to large rather than small or medium-sized companies?
- Would it apply only to those multinational companies using debt-financed models?
- What would be the estimated cost – and opportunity cost – of the compensation associated with any such measure?
- How could continuity of care, stability of provision and protection of the workforce be assured?
- Could it lead to an undue focus on sectoral ownership at the expense of high-quality care?

The CHPI (2019) proposed a gradualist approach whereby the government would make low-cost borrowing available for local authorities to develop a range of home sizes and care models. A decision could then be made about whether to operate these services themselves or outsource day-to-day control to other private or not-for-profit providers. This would also offer protection against the risks associated with the financial collapse of a care home company. A more radical approach was evident in the Labour Party manifesto for the 2019 general election (Labour Party, 2019), which foresaw the public sector once again playing 'the majority role' in delivering adult social care via a National Care Service. Central to this proposal was placing care staff in local authority employment, with enhanced pay, security and working conditions. Given the scale of the defeat of the Labour Party in that election, it remains to be seen whether these arguments have reached their political high point.

Arguably, adult social care is a more problematic sector for renationalisation than others, such as the railways, utility companies or the small probation service. The sector has three complicating features, all of which have been examined elsewhere in this book: penetration, fragmentation and fragility.

Penetration

The provision of adult social care is effectively privatised. Early talk of a 'mixed economy of care', with local authorities, private companies and the voluntary sector competing on a 'level playing field', rapidly evaporated (Wistow et al, 1996). In 1979, 64 per cent of residential and nursing home beds were still provided by local authorities or the NHS; by 2012, it was 6 per cent. In the case of domiciliary care, 95 per cent was directly provided by local authorities as late as 1993; by 2012, it was just 11 per cent (CHPI, 2013). The likelihood is that the longer the period over which outsourcing has taken place, and the greater the penetration of the market, the more difficult it will be to reverse the situation. This is precisely the situation with adult social care, where the process has been in train for over 30 years and the current structure and culture are deeply embedded.

Fragmentation

The sector is characterised by a multiplicity of fragmented, competing providers. The care home sector supports around 410,000 residents across 11,300 homes from 5,500 different providers (Competition and

Markets Authority, 2017), while the situation with home care is even more diverse, with almost 900,000 people receiving help from over 10,000 regulated providers (United Kingdom Home Care Association, 2016). Nor is it any longer the case that the state is even the dominant commissioner of these services. The privatisation of care provision, alongside tighter access to local authority-funded care, has resulted in a rise in self-funding 'customers' accessing support that is exclusively or largely dependent upon their fees – indeed, in some wealthier parts of the country, self-funders constitute the majority of the care market. The sheer size and complexity of this market means that strategies that might work in more simply structured sectors, such as empowering the state to take a foundation share in private companies and appointing non-executive directors to their boards via a public benefit company model, would be difficult to emulate.

Fragility

The third complicating feature of the social care market is fragility – the prospect of significant market failure and the impact of this on highly vulnerable people. As larger operators have begun to populate the sector, the potential for a large-scale market failure, as occurred with Southern Cross in 2011, has increased. The 'hollowed-out' public sector is in no easily attainable position to undertake substantial new roles in care provision (Lobao et al, 2018). In the absence of the restoration of capacity to local government, any move to bring back a substantial part of the sector into public ownership could trigger a damaging departure from the market, with highly problematic consequences for those using services.

None of this is to say that some form of renationalisation or expansion of public sector provision is impossible or undesirable – far from it. However, it would not be a simple task. When the capacity of the state to steer, plan, fund and provide a service has been eaten away over several decades, it cannot easily be restored. Chapter 6 examines the essential context for such a restoration.

Retain and reform the market

Much more attention has been paid to ways in which the dominant market model can be reformed and retained, rather than abolished. These efforts fall into two broad camps: strengthening the 'customer' and shaping the market.

Strengthening the 'customer'

The key tools here are consumer information and consumer protection. In its response to the report of the Competition and Markets Authority (2017) on evidence of malpractice in care homes, the Department of Health and Social Care (2018b) set out the nature of these two approaches. On consumer information, it stated: 'We want informed consumers to drive competition between providers on quality, leading to quality improvement and reduced quality variation across the sector' (Department of Health and Social Care, 2018b). This is also the thrust of a report by the Local Government and Social Care Ombudsman (2019b), which urges providers to offer better advice on such things as: clear upfront information on fees, charges and contracts; accurate and timely billing and invoices; protection of belongings; termination of contracts; care planning; and complaint handling.

On consumer protection, the Department of Health and Social Care said that the government shared the objective of the Competition and Markets Authority to embed consumer law compliance in the sector and that it would strengthen regulations where appropriate and develop model contracts (Department of Health and Social Care, 2018a). The Competition and Markets Authority (2018) itself published further guidance, with four themes: *upfront information* – what should be provided to prospective residents and their representatives; *treating residents fairly* – what should be done to ensure the way residents are fairly treated under consumer law; *quality of service* – how to comply with obligations to perform services to residents with reasonable care and skill; and *complaints handling* – ensuring complaints-handling procedures are easy to find, easy to use and fair.

Successful complaints have been increasing. The Local Government and Social Care Ombudsman (2019a) reported an increase of 16 per cent in 2018/19, with many failings driven by attempts to ration scarce resources. The biggest area of complaint was assessment and care planning, followed by matters related to financial charging. Complaints were also the focus of a report by Independent Age (2019), which – in relation to the different matter of access to care – distinguished between complaints and appeals. Councils have the ability to introduce an appeals process over denial of access to care if they wish but it is not a statutory duty, and only about one in five councils have done so. Most use the statutory complaints system, which can be a slow process taking many months to complete. The report recommends a statutory process that: is distinct from complaints; includes clear provision for an independent reviewer; is clearly explained to individuals; has assigned timescales; includes a requirement to collect data; and is adequately resourced.

There is some evidence of this approach having isolated success. The American-owned care homes group Sunrise Senior Living, for example, agreed to pay £2 million compensation to former residents for having charged them upfront fees (averaging around £3,000) for unclear purposes, and that were non-refundable, after living in one of their homes for more than 30 days. However, for the most part, these sorts of interventions do not reflect what we understand about how people 'consume' care in difficult and fraught circumstances. As McLaughlin (2009), has noted, this discourse assumes that the ideal 'customer' or 'consumer' is one who is able to rationally access services through the market, 'buying' in services in an effective and efficient way to meet their own needs, irrespective of whether the service is provided by the state or the private sector. Individuals are understood as having made a choice in full awareness of the relevant facts and features of their situation, and after a careful analysis of the consequences of each of the choices, selecting the one that is most likely to serve their best interests. Such a view negates how social or personal circumstances impact on individuals' abilities to make rational decisions, especially in the case of those funding their own care with little or no support and often in the heat of an emergency.

Shaping the market

The idea that the market in adult social care can be 'shaped' has reactive and proactive interpretations. The reactive interpretation is that the state, through intelligence gathering and tighter regulation, can try to forestall market failure. The positive interpretation is that the state can also, through local commissioning powers, plan for a stable and responsive provider market.

Reactive market shaping

The prime focus here is on the financial stability of providers and the extent to which a provider might be in such serious financial difficulty that there is a significant prospect of service cessation. The political bargain being struck is that the price of outsourcing (especially to the private sector) is for these companies to open up their balance sheets to state audit (Hudson, 2014). The collapse of Southern Cross in 2011 led to proposals to address market failure in social care. In its consultation on 'market oversight', the Department of Health (2012: para 79) proposed 'stronger requirements on social care providers to disclose information, and for them to have robust plans in place in case they fall into distress'. This, it was said, was to be a 'light-touch approach' that would be 'proportionate, targeted and would support a diverse market of high quality services' (Department of Health, 2012: para 80). Moreover, the government, it was said, would be 'mindful of the sensitivities' and whoever undertook the role 'would have to respect the commercial sensitivity of such information' (Department of Health, 2012: para 106). None of this suggested a very tough approach was in the offing.

In the event, the Care Act 2014 gave this financial oversight role to the regulator – the Care Quality Commission – which is currently tasked with 'overseeing the finances of an estimated 50 to 60 care providers that it is thought would be difficult to replace were they to go out of business' (Care Quality Commission, 2014). In undertaking this role, the Care Quality Commission is expected to: require regular financial and relevant performance information from some providers; disclose early warning of a provider's failure; and seek to ensure a managed and orderly closure of a provider's business if it cannot continue to provide services. In its annual report on the Care Quality Commission, the House of Commons Health Committee (2014) quickly raised doubts about the ability of the Care Quality Commission to do this job and recommended that the task be given to the then health regulator, Monitor. Arguably, the task is one better suited to a financial regulator than one responsible for the quality of care, and in any case, whatever warning signs the Care Quality Commission might identify, it can do little, if anything, to prevent them escalating.

Proactive market shaping

There are two main obligations and opportunities to proactively shape the care provider market. The first – the 'fit and proper person test' – again falls to the regulator, the Care Quality Commission. The assumption behind this proposal is that at least some of the problems of market failure and service withdrawal arise from the capricious behaviour of key individuals, and that this can be countered by undertaking an assessment of their character. In July 2013, the Department of Health (2013) began a consultation on the introduction of 'fit and proper person regulations' for the directors of any organisation registered with the Care Quality Commission and published the feedback in March 2014 (Department of Health, 2014).

The test identifies four 'concerns' about the character of directors: honesty, integrity, competence and capability. To then qualify as a fit and proper person, a director must: not have been responsible for misconduct or mismanagement in the course of any role with a Care Quality Commission provider; be capable of undertaking the position; be of good character; have the qualifications, skills and experience necessary for the role; and not be prohibited from holding the position under existing law. Although the subsequent Care Quality Commission (2014) consultation paper refers to this test as 'a significant restriction', the impact of such a measure on the prospect of company market failure is likely to be small. The test is confined to directors (executive directors, non-executive directors, chairs and trustees), with senior managers and other staff excluded. Certainly, in the case of large national and multinational organisations and investors, it is unlikely that the 'fit and proper person test' will be a serious consideration in their decision-making.

The second obligation – the obligation to shape local markets – falls to local authority commissioners and has already been examined, in part, in Chapter 3. The Care Act 2014 imposed a new 'market-shaping' role on local authorities. Section 5(1) stated that each local authority 'must promote the efficient and effective operation of a market in services for meeting care and support needs', with a view to ensuring that care users have a variety of high-quality providers from which to choose and 'sufficient information to make an informed decision'. In addition, local authorities were given the duty of 'fostering continuous improvement in the quality of such services and the efficiency and effectiveness with which such services are provided and of encouraging innovation in their provision' (Section 5[2]).

These are ostensibly important obligations, but given that councils have had their budgets severely cut by central government over recent years, it is not clear how these are to be achieved or even what they might mean in practice. In terms of the local state as a 'transformer' or 'catalyst' of the adult social care market, there seems to be no strategy to harness the outsourcing of public services to any strategic direction; rather, the end product is simply market diversification and the extension of 'choice'. Therefore, while a 'market-shaping' role formally exists, it is prevented from being implemented by the financial restraints placed on local authorities and the lack of tools available to them to achieve better terms and conditions for care workers, or higher-quality or more stable forms of provision.

Unsurprisingly, some of the early research into market position statements that local authorities are obliged to produce has revealed disappointing findings. In the case of learning disability services, for example, Broadhurst and Landau (2017) concluded that local authorities were not fully engaging in their market-shaping duties, not least due to the lack of recognition that market shaping is a council-wide responsibility and can only be successful if senior officers across councils (and their partners) acknowledge this and are held accountable. Again, Needham et al (2018) identified a lack of consensus as to what market shaping and personalisation meant in practice, as well as highlighting the influence of contextual factors, such as local demographic and socio-economic profiles, the number of self-funders, constraints on public spending, insufficient staffing, weak consumer power, and poor flows of information.

The research undertaken by Needham et al focused on how local authorities had responded to the duty placed on them by the Care Act 2014 to shape social care markets and the requirement to support individual choice and control through 'personalisation'. The team identified four types of local authority market shaping: procurement (high control, weak relationships); managed market (high control, strong relationships); open market (weak control, weak relationships); and partnership (weak control, strong relationships):

- The *procurement approach* was common within residential and home care markets. Here, a dispersed market of providers was often operating, with the local authority setting rigid contract specifications, such as a so-called 'time and task' approach to home care. There was limited engagement and collaboration with providers or other stakeholders, and people's choice of services was limited.
- In the *managed market* approach, local authorities maintain a high level of control over the social care market and develop close relationships with a small number of providers. It is a top-down approach, in that the local authority specifies the service required. As the local authority is working with a smaller number of providers, service users' choice is limited.
- In the *open market approach*, the role of the local authority is to facilitate the interaction between providers and service users but not to set strong controls on market entry or user choice. This model was found in areas where there are high numbers of direct payments and a range of provider options, including personal assistants and micro-enterprises. The case-study sites that had some open market provision commented on the scope for citizens to operate as micro-commissioners.

- In the *partnership approach*, close relationships are developed between local authorities and providers to co-design and develop service provision, with input from other stakeholders, including communities. This was found to be emerging in some local authorities that were taking a strategic long-term and more outcomes-oriented approach to commissioning. This approach requires high-trust relationships over the long term, and the ability to support people holistically through engaging with partners such as health and housing, as well as wider community assets.

The eight case-study local authorities were using combinations of the four approaches in different sub-markets, without necessarily understanding their interdependence, or deliberately trying to progress to other models. The authors conclude that a combination of the open market and partnership models is most likely to achieve the aims of the Care Act to create effective care markets that stimulate provider innovation and diversity in order to offer personalised support to people using services. The procurement and managed market models, in contrast, are more rule-driven and likely to limit scope for diversity and innovation, inhibiting personalised support. Clearly, all of this requires highly skilled commissioners with a deep understanding of current and future market opportunities and options.

Chapter summary

This chapter has looked at two competing perspectives on the ways in which adult social care could be organised and delivered – via the state or through the market. Both are problematic. Renationalisation would have to deal with a number of difficulties, including the cost of requisitioning assets, dealing with potential legal challenges and addressing the deep penetration of private companies and the fragmentation and fragility of the care market. None of these can be adequately addressed while the state (national and local) remains 'hollowed out'.

The alternative route is to look at ways in which the dominant market model can be reformed and retained, rather than abolished. These efforts fall into three broad camps: strengthening the 'customer'; shaping the market; and controlling the providers. The key tools here are consumer information and consumer protection. There is some evidence of these interventions having isolated success, but for the most part, they do not reflect what we understand about how people 'consume' care in difficult and fraught circumstances. Attempts to 'shape the market' have also yet to deliver any real change on the ground.

The analysis in this chapter suggests that little can be expected to change unless two fundamental aspects of the context are addressed: funding and structure. These are the topic of Chapter 6.

6

Context: funding and administration

Introduction

Adult social care cannot be understood in isolation from its wider environment: it functions in accordance with legal requirements; it has, of necessity, relationships with other services, notably, the NHS; it is affected by the wider context of poverty and inequality; and it is shaped by political perceptions of its significance. However, like all policy domains, it requires two prerequisites to be in place: an adequate funding base and effective administrative capacity. Both have been missing in the case of adult social care.

Funding

Inadequate funding is at the heart of policy dilemmas in adult social care. It has two dimensions. First, there is the long-standing squeeze on local government expenditure by central government. This has had the effect of reducing access to services and support for those dependent upon publicly funded care (and other services) and prompting some providers to leave the market. Second, there is the long-running question of finding a long-term solution to the balance of funding responsibility for long-term care between the state, the individual and families.

Local government funding

Around 65 per cent of providers' income comes from care arranged and funded by local authorities, so the level of council funding is essential to the maintenance of the sector (National Audit Office, 2018a). There is, however, no national budget allocation for social care; instead, it is funded through multiple sources, including both public and private funding. Core funding includes support from central government in the form of a revenue support grant (which is not ring-fenced) provided to local authorities, and additional income generated locally through council tax and business rates. Moreover, unlike the NHS, there is no arrangement for funding over multiple years. Planning and investing for the future is impossible when funding streams are left to annual political caprice.

The current policy is that the main plank of central government support (the revenue support grant) should cease by 2020. Local authorities will then having to rely on local business rates and local council tax but will be able to retain 75 per cent of business rates (up from 50 per cent) through the Business Rates Retention Scheme; the piloting of 100 per cent retention is expected in some parts of the country. The idea is that this will incentivise local government to focus on economic growth rather than look to central government for generic grant support. However, poorer areas will be unable to raise much from business rates – business rate revenue per capita in 2018/19 ranged from £940 in London down to £300 in the North East (New Economics Foundation, 2019). Although there will be 'periodic resets' to equalise funding – where money will be moved around between different local authorities to better match funding to need – it is far from clear that this will be sufficient to even compensate for the loss of the revenue support grant, let alone meet the higher levels of need in these more deprived areas.

To this rapidly changing 'core funding' has been added a multiplicity of short-term programmes that have 'topped up' local authority social care budgets at the margins. These have included: the diversion of funds from the New Homes Bonus; the Better Care Fund, whereby central government has transferred some NHS funding to social care; the social care precept, giving local authorities the opportunity to raise additional income between 2016/17 and 2019/20 through an annual rise in council tax each year (by up to 6 per cent over the period); an adult social care support grant worth £240m in 2017/18, distributed according to need; and an Improved Better Care Fund grant paid directly to local authorities (Wenzel et al, 2018). Further amounts to respond to COVID-19 have now been added (see Chapter 8).

These measures have been both inadequate and inequitable. The cuts to local authority funding since 2010 have been immense and unprecedented. Government funding for local authorities fell by almost 50 per cent between 2011 and 2018, notwithstanding growth in demand for key services, notably, adult social care. Councils' spending is increasingly focused on social care services – this now accounts for 57 per cent of all service budgets. To protect adult social care as best they can, councils have cut what they spend on housing, transport, planning, culture, leisure, the voluntary sector and other key services. In the process, the fabric of civic life is pared to a minimum.

Despite attempts to give relative protection to the sector, spending by councils on social care per adult resident fell by 11 per cent in real terms over this period (Phillips and Simpson, 2018). All of this has left a growing 'funding gap' between available resources and estimated need – a gap estimated by the Association of Directors of Adult Social Services (ADASS, 2018) to have reached almost £8 billion by 2020. One-off responses to stave off collapse have now become routine. In 2019, for example, the government announced an additional allocation of £1.5 billion for social care but this had to be shared between adult and children's services. It also assumed all local authorities would increase their standard council tax rates by 2 per cent (the maximum allowed) and increase their social care precept by a further 2 per cent. Meanwhile, no funding was allocated to cover the £220 million needed to pay for the 6 per cent rise in the national minimum and living wages – measures decreed by the government to be in place from April 2020.

In a highly centralised country like England, there is little that local authorities can do to counteract these measures. Local government used to have a huge role in shaping and delivering a beneficial civic life, with responsibilities for swathes of healthcare, police, schooling, fire and rescue, energy, and more. It is now largely marginalised as an independent source of power and legitimacy – of every £1 raised in taxation 91p is controlled and allocated by central government (McGough and Swinney, 2015). This is a degree of centralisation unseen anywhere else in the Western world, leaving legitimate centres of democratic local governance able to do little more than meet statutory duties and invest in pension funds (Skelcher, 2000).

The prime source of independent local finance – council tax – is over 25 years old and was itself a quick-fix solution to the problems associated with Margaret Thatcher's determination to replace domestic rates with the poll tax. The original council tax bands (using 1991 valuations) have never been changed. The consequence is that council tax is deeply regressive – someone living in a home worth £100,000 faces an effective tax rate five times as high as someone living in a million-pound property (Corlett and Gardiner, 2018). This is only part of a wider problem with the inequity of local government funding. Post-industrial cities in the North of England, together with some inner-city London boroughs, have had the deepest cuts to local public services (Gray and Barford, 2018). In the specific case of adult social care, Phillips and Simpson (2018) estimate that, on average, the 30 councils with the highest levels of deprivation made cuts of 17 per cent per person compared to 3 per cent per person in the 30 areas with the lowest levels of deprivation. These effects have been compounded by a lower capacity on the part of councils in deprived areas to mitigate cuts through local taxation or asset sales, and will be exacerbated by plans to phase out central government grants in favour of local business rates.

Local government has become increasingly reliant on local taxes for revenues. Council tax paid by local residents makes up almost half of revenues – up from just over a third in 2009/10 – and retained business rates account for 30 per cent, up from nil (Harris et al, 2019). In desperation, the National Audit Office has reported some English councils resorting to buying office buildings and shopping centres to offset the impact of government funding cuts (National Audit Office, 2020c) – a move that was liable to leave them badly exposed in the event of an economic recession or a property crash – indeed, COVID-19 had exactly that effect. As ever, there is regional variation. Between 2017 and 2020, the more prosperous councils in the South East spent £3.5 billion on such acquisitions compared to £131 million in the North East.

The approach to funding local government contrasts sharply with the way the NHS is funded. The NHS Funding Act, introduced after the 2019 general election, sets out the minimum revenue funding that the NHS will receive every year until 2024, though it does not cover training for doctors, nurses and allied health professionals, or the capital budget. This does allow for some degree of confident forward planning. Local authorities, on the other hand, are unable to plan for services when they do not know what their budget will be, and this soon has knock-on effects to service providers unable to have confirmation of contracts. Indeed, healthcare (a welfare state legacy service) is arguably swallowing up the resource left over for social care (a pre-welfare state means-tested service) – the NHS accounts for about 7 per cent of the economy, compared with 5 per cent for pensions and 1 per cent for adult social care (Smith, 2019).

Over time, these reductions in local government funding have impacted upon access to care and support. The Care Act 2014 introduced a national minimum eligibility threshold (similar to the level of 'substantial' need under the previous 'fair access to care services' criteria) in order to provide some consistency in the way that eligibility is determined in different areas across the country (House of Commons Library, 2020b). In principle, local authorities cannot restrict eligibility beyond the defined threshold; in practice, rules around eligibility are opaque and councils have been able to ration services ever more tightly to remain within their budgets while still apparently adhering to national eligibility criteria.

What then ensues is – as Fox (2018) puts it – resource-starved people and families and resource-starved front-line practitioners both expending time and money they can ill afford on a fruitless battle with each other. At best, a sympathetic assessor might advise people to focus on their 'worst days' rather than identify capacities that could trigger ineligibility. Inevitably, unmet need grows. According to estimates made by Age UK (2018), the numbers of older people in England who struggle without the help they depend on to carry out essential everyday tasks (such as getting out of bed, going to the toilet, washing and getting dressed) increased to a new high of 1.4 million in 2018. This amounted to nearly one in seven older people living with some level of unmet need – a 19 per cent increase over the 2015 estimate. In turn, this increases the demands upon unpaid carers. More families and friends are providing care to relatives and neighbours than ever before – an increase from 4.9 million in 2001 to 5.4 million in 2011, and expected to reach 9 million by 2037 (Carers UK, 2019b).

Funding long-term care

In addition to a sustainable level of funding for local government, there is the long-standing issue of the respective contributions of the individual, the family and the state to the costs of long-term care. The means test that determines these arrangements is stringent. The lower and upper capital limits were increased year on year from 2001/02 to 2010/11 and then frozen since without even an update to reflect inflation. There is a lower means test (set at £14,250) below which individuals are not required to contribute to the cost of their care; there is also an upper means test (set at £23,250) above which individuals are expected to meet the full costs of their care themselves. In the case of residential care, the person's housing assets are taken into consideration as part of the means test, but in the case of domiciliary care, they are not. Moreover, those with assets between £14,250 and £23,250 are still expected to make some contribution to their care, calculated on the basis of £1 per week for every £250 of assets above the £14,250 minimum.

This situation has resulted in the creation of three groups of users with different financial arrangements: those whose income and assets are sufficiently low to qualify for full funding by the local authority; those who pay for the full costs of their care themselves, either because they do not qualify for local authority-funded care, or because they choose not to take it up; and those whose care is funded by a mixture of local authority payments and self-payments, or third-party top-up payments. These top-up payments are made by a third party (typically the person's relatives) when someone chooses to receive care from a provider that charges more than the rate paid by the local authority. The pure market (self-funders) plus the quasi-market (part self-funders who top up) stands at 45 per cent – around the same as the pure local authority-funded group for residential and nursing care.

The history of the past two decades – from the Royal Commission on Long Term Care established in 1997, through multiple green papers, white papers, commissions, reviews and reports – bears testimony to the political intractability of this issue. At the heart of the debate is the ethical question about the balance of responsibility between the state, the individual and families for financing long-term adult social care support. The decision on this principle will determine what the government offers in terms of access, equity, fairness and entitlement to care; it will also determine the scale of public funding required, and the distribution of cost and risk.

Possible approaches range from models in which all, or the vast majority, of care is paid for by the state (generated through taxation), to ones in which people are expected to meet the full costs of their care themselves. There are three broad options for change: adjusting the current 'mixed' system; a social insurance model; or making adult social care free at the point of use.

Adjusting the current system

The minimal adjustment to current arrangements would be to retain the established system but inject some additional funding. The most common suggestion here is to change the funding on caps and floors in order to avoid catastrophic care costs (and avoid the necessity of selling off all assets) and to ease the stringency of the means test. Depending on where the means test is set, it could protect individuals with low wealth against catastrophic costs but those above the floor could still bear high costs unless there was also a cap on lifetime costs. There have been many proposed variations on this theme but the most well known is the Dilnot Report (2011), which proposed, among other things: that individuals' lifetime contributions towards their social care costs should be capped, after which individuals would be eligible for full state support; that this cap should be between £25,000 and £50,000, with £35,000 considered to be the most appropriate and fair figure; and that the means-tested threshold above which people are liable for their full care costs should be increased from £23,250 to £100,000. The Dilnot recommendations were passed into law as Part 2 of the Care

Act 2014 (albeit with a higher cap of £72,000), but after several years of delay in implementation, this part of the legislation was abandoned.

Social insurance/hypothecation model

Social insurance is a common form of hypothecation and is often discussed as an option for funding long-term social care. It is a model that has been adopted in other countries, such as Japan and Germany, and would typically involve contributions from employers, employees and the state, with a significant proportion of contributions coming from wage earners. This approach has advantages. The Japanese and German models look purely at need, whether it arises as a result of physical illness or dementia, with each individual assigned to a support level on a multi-point scale of need. There is no talk of means tests or caps and floors; contributions are clear and paid on a monthly basis out of income or pensions.

The model is also not without problems. First, it is reliant upon a strong economy: if people are out of work, revenue drops and the amounts raised may need topping up. In any case, demand can easily exceed the amount available in the fund and this can lead to unpopular increases in contributions. If opting out is allowed, the scheme may then be able to offer only limited coverage and the likelihood is that those with less ability to pay premiums would be more likely to opt out. A variant on this approach was proposed by the Conservative Party politician Damian Green (2019), involving a universal entitlement to 'basic care needs' supplemented by a voluntary insurance-funded 'top-up' for those wanting a higher level of care. This solution only applies to risks associated with old age. For people of working age, funding cannot be resolved through insurance or a co-payment system – mental illness tends to begin early in life, while learning disability and autism are lifelong conditions. A funding settlement that requires people to save or insure themselves for future risk cannot meet their needs.

As this sort of approach is very different from that taken in the heath sector and in other public services in the UK, introducing it would involve a significant cultural shift (King's Fund, 2018). England has no precedent of social insurance; taxation is a more familiar mechanism that can draw on contributions from income and wealth. In Germany, by contrast, there is a structured and clearly defined framework spanning all ages, with benefits awarded on need alone regardless of age, postcode, diagnosis or living circumstances. This required a major policy shift (moving away from means testing), unlike in England, where a piecemeal approach devoid of fundamental reform has persisted. The narrative in Germany was that long-term care is a social risk rather than an individual risk, and the system should be designed around that principle. In England, there is no such clear narrative or set of principles (Curry et al, 2019).

Free care at the point of use

There is a fundamental lack of alignment between the English health and care systems, in that social care is subject to a needs test and a means test, while healthcare is largely comprehensive and free at the point of use. The underpinning philosophy behind the way in which the NHS is funded is Rawls' (1971) 'veil of ignorance' – the idea that since no one knows if they will be struck down by serious illness, it is therefore in everyone's interests that healthcare is funded by a progressive taxation system to ensure that it is there for us all when we need it. It is a premise that could equally be applied to adult social care.

A host of commissions, inquiries and reports, commencing with the Royal Commission of 1997 (Sutherland Report, 1999), have recommended making social care free at the point of use. Sutherland proposed that personal care should be free but that living costs and housing would be met from people's savings and income, with the means test level raised to £60,000. No action was taken on this or a host of similar subsequent reports. Scotland, however, has operated with this model since 2002, with free personal care provided to anyone aged over 65 on the basis of need, regardless of their level of income or savings and assets. It is important, however, to distinguish between free 'personal care' and free 'social care'. In the case of the former, only some types of social care would be free, for example, help with washing and dressing. This is the system that operates in Scotland, which excludes much social care, including support for lower-level needs, wider support in the community and accommodation costs in care homes (Bottery, 2019). In Scotland, people get only £177 a week towards costs even though average bills are more than £600.

In terms of cost, a report from the Health Foundation and the King's Fund (2018) suggested that free personal care would be no more expensive than investing to restore access to 2009/10 levels – a gap of £7billion by 2020/21 and £14 billion by 2030/31. Resources might be obtained in many ways, including: a small increase in national insurance contributions or on all rates of income tax; the means testing of winter fuel payments; a hypothecated social care tax; the cancellation of the planned reduction in corporation tax from 2020; and reviewing the range of tax reliefs, which had grown to £164 billion by 2018/

19 (Resolution Foundation, 2018). In addition, it has been estimated that the government could gain £90 billion over ten years if it taxed income from wealth in the same way it taxes income from work (Roberts et al, 2019).

Administrative capacity

Any reference to 'public administration' is likely to elicit a yawn, yet it is anything but insignificant; it is the key means by which we put into effect the values, principles and policies that we have collectively decided should shape our lives. It emerged and developed as an alternative mechanism to market or philanthropic endeavour as a means of shaping the allocation of goods and services. However, in the case of local government – the responsible body for organising the local delivery of adult social care – there has never been any comprehensive strategy in England to ensure that it can fulfil administrative purpose (Sanford, 2019b). This situation is in stark contrast to the rest of Europe (Ruano and Profirolu, 2019).

The hollowing out of local government

In the past, following on from the Municipal Corporations Act 1835, local authorities pioneered welfare provision, cleared slums and built houses, parks, hospitals, museums, libraries, swimming pools and playing fields, as well as taking on responsibility for gas, water, electricity and transport. Little is left of this legacy. The financial subjugation of local government to central government has already been noted, and with this fiscal subservience, the creation of the British state as a municipal project has been eroded. Now, the position has been reached where elected local authorities in England are unable to provide and administer many of the features and functions that would normally be expected of a local state.

Since 1945 – and especially in England – the will of central government has been unchecked by any serious form of political devolution. The wave of nationalisation after 1945 was the initial weakening of this tier of government, notably, with the centralisation of the NHS and the transfer of municipal hospitals to central government control. Stewart (2014) suggests that 1974 may have been an important subsequent turning point as functions began to be moved from local government responsibility and given to appointed boards. As the map of local government become increasingly complex, public understanding of where responsibilities for government at the local level lay became reduced. Ministers at the central government level increasingly came to see local authorities as agencies for the provision of services in accordance with national policies, rather than as locally accountable institutions meeting the needs and aspirations of local communities and citizens.

Gamble (1988) warned back in 1988 that the logic of government policy at that time was the eventual abolition of local government. Since then, the establishment of a neoliberal consensus has not just been about creating a new model for the delivery of public services; it has also been an anti-municipal project – an attempt to destroy a potentially rivalrous 'state within a state'. To this end, there has been the marketisation of virtually every aspect of local services – not just adult social care, but children's services, housing and schools, all of them the staple functions of a local tier of governance. This is not normal. Hambleton (2014) undertook a study of 'place-based' leadership in 14 countries and cities, from Copenhagen to Curitiba, Freiburg, Malmo, Melbourne and Portland, and from Denmark to Brazil, Germany, Sweden, Australia and the US. He concluded that with its top-down 'we know best' approach, England is completely out of step with progressive policymaking in other countries.

The lesson drawn by Hambleton was that for England to prosper economically and socially, there needed to be an entirely new strategy for the development of sub-national governance, one that learns from abroad and leads to a significant strengthening of the fiscal and policy power of elected local governments. Much the same conclusion was arrived at more recently by the UK2070 Commission (2020), which found the UK to be one of the most spatially unequal economies in the developed world, with productivity and employment growth concentrated in London and the wider South East. As well as calling for a levelling up of access to funding across the country, the commission also emphasised the need for a comprehensive framework for devolution.

Administrative capacity is necessary for achieving policy success or, at a minimum, avoiding policy failure at the local level. This is problematic when the main delivery body is under existential threat – indeed, in 2018, Northamptonshire County Council actually voted to abolish itself. Although this threat is most evident in the funding reductions described earlier, it also arises from the fact that there is no clarity on the *purpose* of local government in England. In its report into local government spending, the House of Commons Committee of Public Accounts (2019) concluded that the Department for Communities and Local Government (the responsible central government department) had an unacceptable lack of ambition for the sector, with no aspiration beyond merely 'coping'. Not only was it said to have no ambition to improve the financial sustainability of the sector; it did not even know what its minimum expectations were of the full range of services that councils were expected to provide. The question posed in a path-breaking Fabian Society pamphlet by L.J. Sharpe written in 1965 – *Why Local Democracy?* (Sharpe, 1965) – seems to remain unanswered.

This failure to undertake a rational and comprehensive approach to local governance has now resulted in a multiple patchwork of structures at the local, sub-regional and regional levels – some cover traditional local councils; others consist of bigger combined authorities. At the same time, significant powers and budgets have been allocated to influential external bodies, such as local enterprise partnerships (LEPs), the Northern Powerhouse, the Midlands Engine, the Towns Fund and the Future High Streets Fund.

The current central government penchant is for 'metro mayors', which have been established in six areas of England. These have three features in common with earlier models of devolution: limited power over funding; an emphasis on 'soft power'; and minimal engagement with the public. Sanford (2019b) concludes that these bodies pose no real challenge to the balance of power and will simply create more additions to the jumble of bodies making up English local governance. This is a policy approach in which ministers decide the criteria, the contents of each 'deal', what funding will flow to selected areas and even what sort of governance should be in place, regardless of local wishes (Hambleton, 2014). Moreover, attention has been increasingly focused on 'functional economic areas' as a source of local identity – a concept invoked by the 2010 Coalition government to justify the abolition of the nine regional development agencies in favour of LEPs, thereby clashing with historical administrative boundaries.

In the case of adult social care, there have been multiple short-term funding initiatives but no long-term funding plan or strategic direction for the sector. In addition, there is a lack of coordinated monitoring of the impact of funding reductions across the full range of public services, so that while individual government departments may have an understanding of the service areas for which they are accountable, they fail to take account of the implications in other service areas (House of Commons Library, 2020a). Hence, the interdependencies between adult social care, housing, social security and healthcare still remain largely unaddressed. It is in this context that the National Audit Office (2018c) concluded that 'central government needed to build a consensus about the role and significance of local government as a whole'. It is hard to imagine such a recommendation needing to be made in other developed nations.

Joined-up services

Despite – and sometimes because of – the absence of a clear role and accompanying powers for local government, interest has turned to 'joined-up' working across administrative boundaries. Here, the administrative dilemma is that increasingly ambitious policy goals have outstripped the capacity of existing structures and processes to respond. In the case of adult social care, these high-level goals are contained in concepts such as 'well-being', 'independent living'[2] and 'personalised care' – ideas examined further in Chapter 7. Goals such as these require an administrative system capable of focusing beyond the remit of individual organisations. Attempts to address this governance deficit have been twofold: first, a multiplicity of attempts to 'join up' social care with healthcare; and, second, a focus on 'place' rather than organisations.

The most frequent concerns about potential intersections are those with the NHS, where social care is felt to be adversely resulting in delayed transfers of care from hospital, as well as failing to help prevent emergency admissions. The drive from NHS organisations (and also the Department of Health and Social Care) to reduce 'delayed transfers of care' from hospital can too easily translate into the hasty and inappropriate provision of expensive packages of nursing or social care that may be hard to disentangle once implemented. This has led to a situation in which adult social care has been increasingly judged by the extent to which it solves the problems of another organisation, rather than developed as a valued function in its own right (Hudson and Henwood, 2002).

Attempts to join up the two sectors have a long history, one that (in the wake of the purchaser–provider split in both domains) has been characterised by different forms of 'joint commissioning'. There are many reasons for the growing interest in jointly commissioning health and social care, and these are summarised in Table 3.

Hudson (2011b) noted the contrast between the aspirations that arose in the wake of the purchaser–provider split across both policy domains and the relatively limited achievements. The conclusion to emerge from the analysis was that there are severe limits to what can be achieved through top-down, command-and-control systems to encourage joint working. In part, this is caused by ambiguous and conflicting policy messages; however, primarily, it is a model that ignores the de facto

Table 3: Joint commissioning policy imperatives

Efficiency/value for money	Both the NHS and local government are facing huge budgetary reductions. Encouraging them to work together to achieve efficiency through joint commissioning may be one way of coping with this situation.
The 'place' agenda	An emerging policy focus in England is to look at the needs of geographical localities as a whole, rather than working in separate organisations. Joint commissioning could encourage a focus on working together rather than delivering silo-driven, centrally imposed targets.
Personalisation	Personalised support is a key policy objective in England. Individuals' needs rarely fit around traditional service boundaries, especially in the more complex cases. If services are to become more tailored to individual needs, a more coherent approach to support will be required.
Prevention	Prevention is seen as important as a means of driving efficiency and as a policy end in its own right that will improve people's quality of life. To be successful, it will require numerous inputs of services and support that include (but also go beyond) both the NHS and social care.
Care closer to home	The opportunity for improvement created by joint commissioning is to enable more care to be provided closer to home and to reduce the use of expensive and often inappropriate residential and hospital services.
Overlap of clientele	The people who make use of health and social care are often one and the same. In order to ensure a holistic view of their needs, it is essential that their support is jointly planned and commissioned.

Source: Hudson (2011b)

power of front-line professionals, especially clinicians. It is also an approach that views adult social care through the lens of what matters to a different organisation – the NHS – rather than that of people who use or need care support.

None of this has dampened enthusiasm for new initiatives and programmes emanating from the Department of Health and Social Care and NHS England. These include health and wellbeing boards, new models of care, vanguard programmes, sustainability and transformation partnerships, and integrated care systems (House of Commons Health and Social Care Committee, 2018; National Audit Office, 2018b; Visram et al, 2020). Although proclaimed to be seeking to deliver integrated care for vulnerable patients, for the most part, the level of engagement with local government and with adult social care leaders has been weak, and the evidence for success limited (Erskine et al, 2018).

The most recent incarnation is 'primary care networks' (PCNs), intended to cover 30,000–50,000 patients registered with a general practitioner. The Nuffield Trust undertook a 'pre-mortem' exercise to consider the threats and weaknesses of the introduction of PCNs by imagining their hypothetical failure (Edwards and Kumpunan, 2019). Six risks were identified: failure inherent in the policy design; inability to create effective organisations; lack of focus; failures of leadership and followership; becoming overwhelmed by external pressure; and unfair early identification of failure. It would be surprising if the PCN programme avoided all of these pitfalls.

Perhaps surprisingly, the limited success of joint working between these two organisations has not dented aspirations for even more ambitious arrangements, often encapsulated by the notion of 'place-based commissioning'. Here, the policy task is to determine where this 'place' is best located – whether at the regional, sub-regional, local or neighbourhood levels – and to develop an administrative structure capable of ensuring strong organisational coordination at the right level for different tasks. The concept of 'place-shaping' dates from the Redcliffe-Maud Report (Redcliffe-Maud Commission, 1969: 10), which stated that local government's functions should include 'an all round responsibility for the safety, health and wellbeing, both material and cultural, of people within different localities'. The concept was developed further in the Lyons Inquiry (2007), which saw local government as a convenor of the views of the locality on public bodies not under its control.

There has been no shortage of ill-fated attempts to develop 'place-based' approaches. The Blair government embraced a 'new localism', with such initiatives as the New Deal for Communities and Neighbourhood Renewal. The Coalition government of 2010 then introduced the Localism Act 2011, which sought to achieve a substantial and lasting shift in power away from central government and towards local people (Parker, 2015), and followed this up with the ill-fated 'Big Society' initiative (Hudson, 2011a). By 2017, the Institute for Government (Wilson et al, 2017) had identified around 60 government initiatives aimed at reducing 'silos' since 1997, such as Total Place, Our Place and the Troubled Families initiative, none of which could be said to have achieved notable success.

Chapter summary

Adult social care, like any other policy domain, requires an adequate funding base and effective administrative capacity in order to function successfully. This chapter has argued that both of these essential building blocks are absent. While there are many different proposals for change, and much lively debate about various models for delivery, these will amount to little until the funding and administration problems are addressed.

Inadequate funding is at the heart of policy dilemmas in adult social care. It has two dimensions: first, there is the long-standing squeeze on local government expenditure by central government; and, second, there is the long-running question of settling a long-term solution to the balance of funding responsibility for long-term care between the state, the individual and families. Meanwhile, there has been a total neglect of 'public administration' – the key means by which we put into effect the values, principles and policies that we have collectively decided should shape our lives.

In the case of local government – the responsible body for organising the local delivery of adult social care – there has never been any comprehensive strategy in England to ensure that it can fulfil administrative purposes. This has now resulted in a multiple patchwork of structures at the local, sub-regional and regional levels, with ministers at the central government level increasingly having come to see local authorities merely as agencies for the provision of services in accordance with national policies, rather than as locally accountable institutions meeting the needs and aspirations of local communities and citizens.

7

Looking ahead: an ethical future for adult social care

Ethics and ethical care

In his classic work *The Language of Morals*, the philosopher R.M. Hare (1952) argued that a 'moral statement' is one that prescribes a course of action – it is recommending that something *should* be done rather than just expressing the feelings of the speaker. Ethics is therefore about how human beings should treat each other, and it covers matters of rights, responsibilities and well-being. However, ethics is not only about finding the right response to a given dilemma; it is also about justifying the decisions and choices made. According to well-established theories, actions can be judged as right or wrong according to either their consequences (as in *utilitarian theories*) or according to conformity to ethical rules or duties (as in *deontological theory*). A further position is '*virtue ethics*', which holds that it is *the character* of the moral agent that matters – a good person performs good actions, which have been learned and acquired through experience, practice, role models and good examples (Rachels and Rachels, 2015).

Regardless of the theoretical stance, ethics has to be capable of application to practical situations. This was the Victorian tradition, for example, with Bentham's concern with prison reform and J.S. Mill's campaign for women's suffrage. More recently, the interest has focused on defining the place of ethical behaviour in professional responsibilities – about how people in professional roles ought to behave. Banks (2012), for example, identifies three clusters of complex values that should guide professional behaviour, all of them germane to adult social care:

- *respect for the dignity and worth of all human beings* – respect each human being as an individual, treat all people as equally valuable and respect the right to self-determination;
- *promotion of welfare or well-being* – the obligation to bring about benefits for service users and for society more generally; and
- *promotion of social justice* – the obligation to remove damaging inequalities.

The literature on the 'ethics of care' focuses on the responsibilities inherent in situations where individuals are defined in terms of their relationships with others. For Held (2006), this involves valuing rather than rejecting emotion – sympathy, empathy, sensitivity and responsiveness are the sorts of emotions that need to be cultivated. Tronto (2010) distinguishes between four aspects of care:

- *caring about* – recognising a need for care;
- *caring for* – taking responsibility to meet that need;
- *care giving* – the actual physical work of providing care; and
- *care receiving* – understanding how well the care provided has met the caring need.

It would be a mistake, however, to confine ethics and ethical behaviour to front-line practice; rather, it applies equally to all of those involved in public life, to politicians, policymakers, managers and owners of private companies in receipt of public monies. Minstrom (2010), for example, proposes five principles of 'moral competence in public life':

- *Integrity*: when people act with integrity, they are directed by an internal moral compass – they strive to do the right thing in any given situation and to achieve consistency in their intentions and actions across contexts. This is the foundation for living an ethical life – the following of high standards of honesty, alongside a commitment to the values of justice and fairness.
- *Competence*: a strong relationship exists between competence and ethical behaviour – it is dishonest for anyone to say that they can do something when they cannot.
- *Responsibility*: taking responsibility means acknowledging the part you play in contributing to outcomes – it is commonplace for people to willingly accept the credit when good outcomes occur but to deflect blame for poor outcomes.
- *Respect*: when we show respect for others, we acknowledge their humanity, dignity and right to be the people they are. It means being considerate and appreciative of others – treating others as you would like to be treated.
- *Concern*: living an ethical life requires that we show concern for others and not just for those who are close family members or friends – it means caring about, showing an interest in and being involved in the lives of others.

It is reasonable to expect all of those involved with, and working in, adult social care to be active moral agents, guided by ethical principles and making a critical interpretation of relevant ethical codes. However, as noted earlier, Unwin (2018) suggests that kindness, emotion and human relationships can too easily become the 'blind spot' in public policy. Indeed, she points out that kindness can be a double-edged sword as it is frequently associated with a patronising and pitying approach – something that will be strongly resisted by those committed to a culture of rights and entitlement.

In the case of social work (as opposed to the more generic 'social care'), ethical principles for professional practice have been developed. The ethical code of the British Association of Social Workers (2012) refers to promoting dignity, well-being and self-determination, attending to the whole person, identifying and building strengths, challenging discrimination, recognising diversity, distributing resources, and working in solidarity. All practitioners, it is said, should aim to uphold these principles. Again, British Association of Social Workers (2019) guidance on anti-poverty practice urges social workers to focus their practice on promoting income maximisation and the full take-up of benefit entitlements, and working with food banks. Practitioners are also urged to evidence how poverty is leading to a denial of people's rights – a stance that resonates with the 'radical social work' model of past decades.

Where a recognised and regulated profession – like medicine, nursing or social work – is responsible for delivering a service, then ethical behaviour might be expected to be a central feature, with breaches of ethical codes leading to loss of a licence to practise. Things become murkier when the bulk of provision is privatised to over 20,000 companies and those working in the sector do not belong to an occupation holding professional status. However, the picture is bigger than just those working at the front line; it is also a matter of ethical public policy.

Government handles morality as of necessity; it is the very stuff of its existence. Yet, as Henricson (2016) notes, politicians like to segregate the moral sphere from core public policy and hive it off as the provenance of private conscience. This is a false division: public policies are about what governments choose to do (or choose not to do) and what principles should guide their decision-making. In this sense, ethics lies at the heart of public policy and all aspects of the policymaking cycle – defining the problem, identifying and assessing the available options, decision-making, implementation, evaluation and termination. Ethical neutrality by the state is not an option.

The philosopher Bernard Williams argues that the important question is not 'what is the best form of society', but rather 'what is the best form of society we can get to, starting from here?' (Williams, 2005: 23). Taking where we currently are with adult social care as our starting point – that is, the positions described in Chapter 2, the dilemmas examined in Chapters 3 and 4, and the context explored in Chapter 5 – how can an ethical focus be articulated and incorporated into adult social care commissioning? Four suggestions are made here:

- commissioning ethical employment practice
- commissioning for well-being
- commissioning local and small
- commissioning personally

Commissioning ethical employment practice

The concept of 'business ethics' is slippery but generally refers to a core set of questions about how individuals in the business world ought to behave, or what set of principles they might appeal to in order to negotiate moral dilemmas arising from business activity (Moriarty, 2017). Three models are generally identified:

- *Stockholder theory*: the stockholders contribute capital to the business and appoint corporate managers who act as agents in advancing stockholder interests. The only social responsibility of business is to use the resources to engage in activities to increase profits for the stockholders.
- *Stakeholder theory*: a stakeholder in any organisation is any group or individual who can affect or is affected by the achievement of the organisation's objectives. Agents are therefore responsible for taking care of all such interests – employees, suppliers, distributors, customers and the local community.
- *Social contract theory*: here, agents are responsible for taking care of the needs of society; such contracts would permit the creation of organisations on the condition that they create more value to society than they consume for their business interactions.

These models are not without resonance in adult social care. Chapter 4 has shown that some of the large providers tend towards stockholder theory, though many others make some attempt to embrace elements of the stakeholder model. Relatively little thought has been given to how adult social care could be framed within the social contract theory perspective. This chapter considers ways in which this might be developed.

The existence of these different models is a reflection of company law, which is something that is changing and could be further changed by legislative intervention. One means of doing so is to look at the ways in which customers, employees and communities can have a say and a stake in how things are run (Cooperative Party, 2018). Commissioning local authorities could use their powers to foster the development of public services contractors that not only respond to the needs of communities, but also empower them through agency, ownership and control – indeed, the public sector should arguably *only* work with providers that can do this. The IPPR's Commission on Economic Justice (IPPR, 2018a), for example, suggests that companies with more than 250 employees should have at least two elected workers on both the main board and the remuneration committee. The report points out that this is not especially radical: in 13 European countries (including Germany, France, Ireland and the Netherlands), workers have significant rights of representation in the private sector.

The idea that a company's only true allegiance should be to its shareholders fails to reflect the relative risks of those with a legitimate interest. Shareholders, especially when they are fund managers, are an ever-changing cast with diversified risks and no fear of bankruptcy. Workers, on the other hand, have livelihoods at stake, and users and carers have support arrangements that could be put in jeopardy. One way of addressing this deficit is changing the Companies Act to redefine a company's responsibilities beyond the promotion of shareholder interests. Corporations in the UK were originally established with clear public purposes; it is only over the last half-century that the corporate purpose has come to be equated solely with profit and the primacy of shareholder interest. A re-conceptualisation of the corporation around social purpose and mission is therefore long overdue. A report from the British Academy (2018), for example, argues the case for replacing property rights views of ownership with one rooted in a redefined corporate purpose within which companies are expected to perform significant social functions.

All of this implies significantly different structures of governance that would include direct workers, service users and citizens. Those companies undertaking significant social functions – and adult social care provision is a prime example – should be among those *most* expected to incorporate public purposes in their corporate purposes. In relation to adult social care, the broad aim would be move the awarding of contracts away from companies with a stockholder ethic and towards those able to demonstrate stakeholder and social contract approaches.

Given that the single biggest cost in adult social care provision is staffing, the prime test of such a shift would be the ways in which the workforce is treated, and this requires action at both the national and local levels. Priority could be given locally to those providers able to demonstrate a commitment to a range of 'good employer' obligations relating to pay and security. At the same time, national government could take serious action on issues related to status, workforce quality and regulation.

Action on pay

As has already been established in Chapter 4, employment in adult social care is characterised by endemic low pay; therefore, the first goal of ethical employment practice would be to correct this situation. Payment of the National Living Wage is often seen as a vital initial measure. The Living Wage Foundation is an accreditation scheme for employers who pay more than the statutory minimum wage by committing to an amount calculated to meet the actual costs of living. In England, around a quarter of local authorities have acquired this accreditation but many of them fail to make the same requirement of their suppliers – a major failing in adult social care, where almost all provision is by external suppliers. Elsewhere in the UK, a stronger line is taken. In Scotland, for example, the Scottish government has offered additional funding for local authorities conditional upon them successfully negotiating a pay rise for care workers in their area that meets at least the level of the real living wage (Alton, 2016).

Given the size of the sector and the endemic levels of low pay, the widespread introduction of the real living wage in social care would not be cheap. The IPPR (2018b) has attempted to estimate the potential costs associated with increasing pay to at least the living wage in social care. Based on pay levels in the sector in 2018, it was calculated that the additional costs of increasing pay in social care to the living wage would be £645 million. In its general report in 2019, the Trade Union Council (2019) took the view that the best way to raise wages and improve conditions was by increasing the number of workers covered by collective bargaining. It the report, it calls for: unions to have rights of access to all workplaces to tell workers about the benefits of membership; new rights to make it easier for working people to negotiate collectively with their employers on issues that go beyond pay, such as workload and family-friendly rights; and sectoral collective bargaining, which would involve the creation of new mandatory joint bodies for unions and employers to negotiate pay, conditions and training for all employees working in a specific sector. Moreover, this process, the report argues, should *start* with adult social care.

Action on security

National action on security could cover the right to a fixed-hours contract and stronger protections for those workers who choose zero-hours contracts – the IPPR (2018a), for example, suggests that the minimum wage should be set 20 per cent higher for those on zero-hours contracts in order to discourage their use and to ensure workers are compensated for greater insecurity. This is not an issue confined to England; for European trade unions as well, one of the most important pledges to emerge from the European Pillar of Social Rights (European Commission, 2017) was a commitment to reinforce workers' legal security. The measures proposed include: a requirement on employers to supply written details of the employment relationship on the first day of work; the ending of unfair terms in contracts, such as long probation periods; stopping workers on flexible contracts having their hours cut back; and the protection of trade union workplace representatives. The application of these measures to England now it has left the EU is unclear.

Action on status

Several options exist to enhance the current low status of adult social care employment. First, professional registration and regulation could be strengthened. A national requirement for care work to become a regulated profession under the Health and Care Professionals Council (the professional registration body) would enhance occupational status by requiring the acquisition of a relevant qualification, setting high standards of conduct and expertise, and debarring those unable to meet these standards from practise. At a minimum, the existing Care Certificate should become a robust and mandatory licence to practise for all care workers. However, there do remain concerns among those who employ their own personal assistants that compulsory registration could take away their choice to employ people who may lack conventional attributes.

England now stands on its own in its absence of a coherent approach to regulation of the social care workforce within the UK. The Scottish social care workforce has been regulated for a number of years by the

Scottish Social Services Council – the final tranche took place at the end of 2019, with all home care and supported housing staff having to register. Wales introduced a system more recently, administered by Social Care Wales, and this was due to be completed (with the registration of domiciliary care workers) by April 2020. Northern Ireland includes the partial registration of the workforce, with the Northern Ireland Social Care Council focusing on the regulation of managers in care homes and domiciliary settings. The situation in England looks completely out of step.

A further means of enhancing professional status would be the creation of a national organisation to represent the interests of care workers, raise the status of their work and promote the importance of their role. Such an organisation could link in to new arrangements on registration, training and continuing professional development, and develop 'portable' certification that could be used across the sector. A development of this kind could perform several roles: ensuring that care workers have an effective voice in the design, development and delivery of services; agreeing minimum contract standards for the provision of publicly funded services, covering pay, hours, security, supervision, training and development; and instigating a radical overhaul of commissioning practices to ensure fair work drives service delivery (Fair Work Convention, 2019). All of this needs to lead into a clearer path for career progression. As is the case with the NHS, pay scales in adult social care should include increments in order to reflect increasing experience and expertise, as well as to give workers greater opportunity for pay progression and greater incentives to stay in the profession.

The All-Party Parliamentary Group on Social Care (2019) undertook an inquiry into ways to 'elevate' the status of those working in adult social care. It called for the immediate formation of a national programme of work to plan and develop a workforce strategy for England, establishing a new identifiable national care body with a bespoke identity, equal status with NHS staff and a new framework of governance, accreditation and leadership. It also called for 'all sectoral stakeholders, policy-makers and politicians to commit now to the elevation of the multi-faceted, complex, increasingly highly skilled social care workforce up to NHS parity' (All-Party Parliamentary Group on Social Care, 2019: 13). Some take the view that this might require unhitching adult social care from the NHS by creating a separate Department of Social Care, Social Care Training Council, Social Care Inspectorate and Social Care Enterprise Agency (Jackson, 2018). Less radically, it could involve reviewing the role of Social Work England

and creating a Royal College of Care Work to match those already in place for GPs, nurses, pharmacists and others.

Action on quality

The trade union Unison (2017a) has developed a 'care charter' that has attracted support from a growing number of local authority commissioners. This goes beyond pay to include such elements as: entitlement to basic induction training and ongoing continual professional development; minimum qualification levels for given roles; minimum requirements for apprenticeship investment and standards; and the right to a fixed-hours contract and protections for workers who choose zero-hours contracts. Again, unlike England, other parts of the UK already take a stronger approach to these matters. The Welsh government launched a Code of Practice on Ethical Employment in Supply Chains in 2017, which covered issues of modern slavery and human rights abuses, blacklisting, false self-employment, zero-hours contracts and paying the living wage. The Procurement Reform (Scotland) Act 2014 goes further in requiring all public bodies to have a procurement strategy in place that supports community benefits, the living wage and the economic, social and environmental well-being of the local area.

Other work suggests that there are advantages to be gained from a 'values-based' approach to recruiting – one in which greater attempts are made to determine whether or not candidates hold the right ethical values, rather than if they can navigate personality profiling tools. This could include, for example, values-based questions and follow-up discussions to reflect on candidates' answers and their application to real situations. One study using data from 112 social care organisations concluded that staff recruited in this way performed better in terms of sickness absence, punctuality and retention (Consilium and Skills for Care, 2016).

Action on regulation and legislation

There could be an important new role here for the regulator, the Care Quality Commission. Given the widespread evidence of poor and often illegal employment practices, and given the link between job quality and care quality, the remit of the Care Quality Commission could be expanded to cover two new duties: a duty to enforce minimum standards in the sector by requiring employers to demonstrate that they have a sufficiently trained workforce, including compliance with the

Care Certificate; and a duty to tackle the exploitation of low-paid care workers, including reporting on non-payment of the minimum wage.

Others propose more far-reaching measures to combat unethical business behaviour. It is currently impossible to know how much of the money going into private care home companies finds its way to the front line rather than dividends to investors. To combat this, the CHPI (2019) has called for a Care Home Transparency Act, mandating providers of adult social care to disclose where their income goes. This would resemble the American Nursing Home Transparency and Improvement Act 2009, which requires nursing homes in receipt of public funding to report details of ownership, staffing levels, other costs, complaints and expenditure categories.

These measures could go further to prevent companies with unsatisfactory financial models from providing care – notably, those that have levered high levels of debt, pay large 'management fees' and are registered outside the UK for tax purposes. Some minimal recognition of this sort of action arose during the COVID-19 outbreak, when the government banned access to its bailout loan schemes to companies paying shareholder dividends, as well as restricting bonus payments to board directors.

Commissioning for well-being

If the pursuit of more ethical employment practices takes adult social care from the 'stockholder' to the 'stakeholder' box, ideas around commissioning for well-being are more focused on the social contract approach. Ideas about 'well-being' are much broader than those around workforce improvements and are correspondingly more difficult to pin down. As noted in a publication from the Local Government Association (2020a), although understanding of the concept will be personal to each of us, some common themes do emerge: family and friendships; hobbies and interests; new experiences; and work and volunteering. All of these things 'connect us to ourselves, to those around us and to the places in which we live' (Local Government Association, 2020a: 4).

Adult social care should be an important part of a well-being strategy. The promotion of well-being is central to the Care Act 2014, where it is described as relating to the following areas in particular: personal dignity (including treatment of the individual with respect); physical and mental health, as well as emotional well-being; protection from abuse and neglect; control by the individual over their day-to-day life (including over care and support provided, as well as the way they are provided); participation in work, education, training or recreation; social and economic well-being; domestic, family and personal domains; suitability of the individual's living accommodation; and the individual's contribution to society (Department of Health and Social Care, 2018b).

This amounts to a formidable mission. Although the introduction of the Care Act made this way of working a statutory duty, it is far from clear that much has been achieved at a time of deep cuts to funding and levels of support (Barnes et al, 2017). A consultation paper from the British Association of Social Workers (2019) further claimed that the Care Act's duty on councils to promote individuals' well-being did not provide a sufficiently clear vision for what social care should achieve, and that it required a standard of well-being against which needs should be measured. This, it was argued, should be consistent with the definition of independent living set out in the United Nations Convention on the Rights of Persons with Disabilities – one that the UK has agreed to follow but that has not yet been incorporated into UK law. The convention states that disabled people should have: the opportunity to live where and with whom they want on an equal basis with others, without being obliged to live in a particular arrangement; access to a range of support services to promote inclusion and prevent isolation; and access to general community services on an equal basis to other people and in a way that is responsive to their needs.

A concept like well-being goes beyond adult social care, where the focus has tended to be upon the individual rather than on a wider sense of 'place'. There is no doubt that the lives of those requiring some form of support are shaped by wider policy domains (especially health, social security and housing) and wider policies, notably, that of austerity (Rahman, 2018). Consideration of these domains is largely beyond the scope of this book, but at the local level, perhaps the most important opportunity to incorporate some version of well-being into public policy has been through the Public Services (Social Value) Act 2012, which 'enables' public sector local authorities to consider wider social, economic and environmental benefits through their procurement procedures.

Even though this is only a discretionary power, in principle, it could be used in social care commissioning processes. There is little evidence that this is happening. Only around a quarter of local authorities seem to have a social value strategy, though a third claims to routinely consider it in their procurement and commissioning; furthermore, even when utilised, social value considerations only amount to between 5 and 10 per cent of contract scoring systems (Social Enterprise, 2016). Nevertheless, it is at the local, rather than central, level where any progress is likely to be made. An investigation by Tussell (2020) found that local government is considerably better at awarding contracts to small and medium-sized enterprises and the voluntary and community sector. In 2018/19, local government awarded contracts to these providers worth £3.9 billion (16 per cent of the value of all of their contracts), compared with £3 billion from central government (6 per cent of total contract value). In addition, local authorities awarded £4.4 billion worth of their contracts to organisations based in their local areas.

There have been calls to extend the Act, and in 2018, the government published its *Civil Society Strategy* (HM Government, 2018), in which it stated that it aspired to strengthen and extend the Act in several ways:

- by applying it to the whole of government spending, including goods and works as well as services;
- by replacing the obligation to 'consider' with a requirement to 'account for' the social value of new procurements;
- by exploring its application in grants as well as contracts; and
- by considering its extension to other areas of public decision-making, such as planning and community asset transfer.

There has been no noticeable progress to date on even these modest aspirations. In the meantime, others have put the case for a more fundamental reworking of the concept and how it can be measured. The Centre for Local Economic Strategies (2018), for example, argues that the Social Value Act should be amended or potentially replaced with a Public Values Act, whereby the right to deliver public services would be dependent on the discharge of clear economic and social obligations, including those concerning workforce issues. In a similar vein, the New Local Government Network (2018) has called for replacing 'social value' with 'social impact' and having a sharper focus on measurable outcomes built into contract management.

Defining and developing the metrics for such interventions is work in progress. One of the areas making most progress – the Greater Manchester Combined Authority – requires bids for tenders to articulate how they will: promote employment and economic sustainability; raise living standards of local residents; promote participation and citizen engagement; build the capacity and sustainability of the voluntary sector through practical support for local voluntary and community groups; provide support for those in the greatest need or facing the greatest disadvantage, as well as tackle deprivation; and promote environmental sustainability. These requirements carry weightings of up to 20 per cent in determining the award of contracts (Local Government Association, 2017).

Policy in Wales appears to be ahead of that in England. Here, the Wellbeing of Future Generations Act (Welsh Government, 2015) requires all public organisations to take into account the long-term effects of any decision they make, as well as the knock-on impact it may have in terms of the prosperity of people in Wales and its environment, culture and communities. Public service boards have been set up for every local authority in Wales, which have to include representatives from the local council, health board, fire and rescue authority, and National Resources Wales, along with an option to also involve services such as probation and voluntary groups. These boards have to publish a local 'well-being plan' and explain how that will lead towards goals set in the Act.

Passing legislation like this is arguably the easy bit. Early evaluation findings on the Welsh legislation reveal the gap that can quickly open up between policy and implementation (Rees et al, 2017). This interim evaluation looked at early attempts to secure more meaningful engagement and involvement with social enterprise, cooperative, user-led and third sector organisations (as set out in the Act), as well as the implementation role of regional partnership boards (RPBs) and regional social value (RSV) forums. It identified a number of implementation threats:

- The absence of a shared understanding of the definition of 'social value' created confusion over what is a 'social value organisation'.
- Austerity placed budgets on the floor, with little room for forward-looking. There was a lack of capacity to deliver transformational change.
- Aversion to risk obstructed the ability to implement change. A lack of internal expertise on social value led to a focus on further information gathering rather than action.
- There was confusion in the relationship between new structural arrangements and existing organisations.
- There was highly variable involvement of the third sector in RPBs. The usual third sector networks do not necessarily encompass social enterprises and cooperatives.
- There was limited impetus to deliver services through more innovative care models. Short-term funding and annual contracts hampered the recruitment and retention of staff.

- There was a lack of clarity on measuring success, reporting and being held to account.

Overall, the challenges were too great, not least due to an environment of competing priorities and adversity to risk. Without start-up funding, social value organisations were finding it impossible to consider new ways of delivering care and support while still managing people 'coming through the front door'. It is a small but important reminder that policy – especially policy seeking to be in some way 'transformative' – requires a policy support programme. This will be considered more in Chapter 9.

Oversight of progress in Wales is undertaken by a Future Generations Commissioner but the role lacks the power to stop things happening or to make things happen – it is essentially a 'name and shame' role. A stronger model of commissioning for well-being seems to be in place in New Zealand, where the government seeks to be the first country to design its entire budget around well-being priorities – initially, child poverty, domestic violence and mental health are the selected domains. The annual budget policy statement has set out how the government is planning to make progress on these issues through the budget while meeting rules on budget responsibility (Deloitte-NZ, 2018). Similar sorts of proposals are being made in the UK, for example, by the All-Party Parliamentary Group on Wellbeing Economics (2019), but progress is still very limited. Overall, the move towards a 'social contract' model is barely out of the blocks.

Commissioning local and small

The dominant trend in adult social care commissioning is one of increasing size – larger-scale provision in the hands of large provider companies. Much of this occurs beneath the public radar, such as bringing together sets of smaller contracts into large single-tender opportunities that favour larger bidders. Similarly, prequalifying questionnaires can be littered with pass or fail questions that undo a prospective bid from smaller organisations. Although many local authorities are signed up to a local compact with the voluntary sector, when it comes to challenging a procurement decision, this will tend to have little force (Newcastle Council for Voluntary Service, 2018). Alongside the commissioning preference for large providers, there is the move among providers themselves towards larger-scale operations, especially in the care home sector. Here the trend is for small-scale operators to be replaced by large provider chains with more than 50 care homes. Industry estimates (Knight Frank, 2019) indicate that as care homes grow in size, they become more profitable, with the highest margin on those with over a hundred beds.

There is evidence to suggest that those on the receiving end of services and support prefer a model that operates at what Fox (2018) calls a 'human scale' and that the people most likely to design these are front-line workers and the people and communities with whom they work. Needham (2014), for example, established that micro-providers were better at delivering personalised domiciliary care because of the increased autonomy given to care staff compared to large providers. More broadly, there is evidence from the Care Quality Commission (2017a) that smaller facilities tend to receive better ratings for quality of care.

This implies the need to look afresh at the potential roles that could be played by 'civil society' in its widest sense – informal networks, community groups, cooperatives, registered charities, social enterprises and a hybrid of all of these forms. However, the evidence suggests that this is largely a sector in disarray due to increased competition for grants and contracts, cuts in spending, an inability to diversify income streams, and a growing demand for services. The Unwin Inquiry (2018) into the sector found it to be lacking in confidence, skills and credibility, while an annual survey of 686 local charities in 2018 found just 47 per cent confident of surviving beyond five years (Localgiving, 2018).

At the same time, 'neighbouring' has been weakening. Almost everyone has neighbours, yet the neighbourhood is a relatively neglected level of analysis – the bulk of academic and policy attention has focused upon the levels *above* the neighbourhood (the political, economic and value systems of society as a whole) or *beneath* it (interpersonal relationships in settings such as the family). However, neighbourhoods derive significance from their proximate status, as compared with the remoteness of other systems of governance, production or consumption; neighbourhoods *do* matter for the people who live in them (Pierson, 2008; Onward, 2020).

After years of political neglect, there are now widespread concerns that public spaces are disappearing, civic institutions are decaying and social relationships are fragmenting. Klinenberg (2018) argues that when social infrastructure is ripped out, people reduce the time they spend in public settings and stay at home. Official figures on social capital in the UK from the Office of National Statistics (2020b) evidence that the sense of belonging to a community has declined in several ways over recent years, for example, a decline in doing favours, stopping to talk and joining political, voluntary, professional and recreational organisations. As social networks weaken, crime rises, older and sick people grow isolated, distrust rises, and civic participation wanes. This wider context is critical to the situation of adult social care. It also turned out to be critical in responding to COVID-19, as will be examined in Chapter 8.

Calls for an alternative approach seeking to revive local relationships are often rooted in some version of the concept of co-production, albeit that this is a slippery concept. Needham and Carr (2009), for example, distinguish between three different levels of co-production. First, there is *basic co-production*, which recognises that while people are inevitably participating in many public services, they may not have any influence on how these services are designed or delivered. Second, there is *intermediate co-production*, which more actively recognises that people using services have skills to offer. This level of co-production means that services recognise and support people's contributions and ideas for improvement but only for helping to deliver services. Finally, *transformational co-production* means that power and control changes, so that people who use services are actively involved in all aspects of designing, commissioning and delivering services.

There is an increasing emphasis on empowering citizens or service users in some way; however, while there has been an explosion of participation initiatives, power rarely seems to be ceded by the organisations concerned. In the case of adult social care, ideas about empowering those who need support have a long history with user-led organisations (ULOs) and disabled people's organisations (DPOs). The roots of both can be traced as far back as the 1960s and the civil rights movements, with the first centre for independent living being set up in Hampshire in 1984. As noted earlier, this movement led the successful campaign for direct payments in social care, culminating in the Community Care (Direct Payments) Act 1996, and was also instrumental in the use of disabled people managing their own care and staff (Evans, 2003). The policy nadir of this movement was probably a publication by the Prime Minister's Strategy Unit (2005), which made a recommendation that every local authority should have an organisation run and controlled by disabled people in place by 2010. This commitment was repeated in the Independent Living Strategy (Office for Disability Issues, 2008). It is far from clear how much progress was made with these ambitions but there has been a loss of focus and there is now no statutory requirement on public bodies to engage with or fund user-led groups in England.

Despite all of these difficulties, there is new evidence of successful community enterprises, ranging from micro-providers delivering support to a handful of people, to community businesses delivering multiple activities for many local people (NDTI, 2020). Many examples have been reported by the organisation Social Care Futures (2019), which argues for a new community-based paradigm in adult social care. These include established models such as Local Area Coordination (Broad, 2012) and Shared Lives (Fox, 2018), newer micro-enterprises like Community Catalysts (2018), and the growth of community businesses encouraged by the lottery-funded charity Power to Change (Bedford and Harper, 2018). Brief summaries of some of these initiatives are as follows:

- *Local Area Coordination*, which originated in Western Australia, is a practical, asset-based approach that is being adopted by a growing number of local authorities and health partners across England, Scotland and Wales. Each local area coordinator works with a defined neighbourhood of 8,000–12,000. These coordinators approach, or are introduced to, people who may be isolated, may be causing concern or are at risk of needing formal services. Coordinators support people to build their own vision for a good life, finding pragmatic solutions to any problems, and drawing on family and community resources, before considering an approach to commissioned or statutory services.
- *Shared Lives* is a membership body that trains potential carers (ordinary people in the community) and matches them with adults who need support. Paid carers welcome elderly people and those with learning difficulties, physical disabilities and mental health issues into their families or communities, and often into their home, as an alternative to traditional care services in residential institutions. Around 9,000 Shared Lives volunteers are now supporting more than 13,000 vulnerable adults across the UK. There is evidence to suggest that this saves significant money for local authorities – an estimated £26,000 a year compared to the cost of residential care (Nesta and SCIE, 2019). More importantly, the model has been shown to deliver better outcomes for the adults accessing the support, for example, with regard to social isolation and loneliness.
- *Community Catalysts* arose as a response to problems in the home care market, which has been finding itself unable to build in time for dignity and companionship. The approach is based on releasing local people's capacity to care by using a 'catalyst' to support around a hundred small, self-organising enterprises over a two-year period. This aim is to create reliable, flexible and personal care for older

people and their families, as well as appropriately paid and highly satisfying self-employment for local people. The programme has supported the development of more than 3,000 community enterprises in over 60 areas of the UK, which support about 14,000 people. There is a particular presence in the South West of England, reflecting the rapidity with which they have developed in Somerset, where they are on course to have around 600 micro-enterprises up and running in 2020.

- *Power to Change* is a Charitable Trust operating in England, having been created in 2015 with a £150 million endowment from the Big Lottery Fund. The trust is solely concerned with supporting community businesses over a ten-year period, after which it will cease operating. The ultimate goal is for the funding to lead to 'better places through community business', reflecting the belief that community businesses contribute more than just economic impact; they can also lead to more community cohesion and a greater appetite for community-led development.

- *The Buurtzorg model* ('*Buurtzorg*' translates as 'neighbourhood care') is famous for pioneering an innovative approach to domiciliary care in the Netherlands. The social enterprise was founded in 2006 by a small group of nurses who were frustrated by reforms that undermined their ability to build relationships with the people they were supporting. Since then, it has grown quickly, taking on more than 3,000 of the workers who lost their jobs when the Netherlands' largest private domiciliary care provider went bankrupt in 2016. It now employs more than 10,000 district nurses, who work in small, self-managing teams and have the autonomy to genuinely co-create support with the people they help. These successes have inspired similar approaches in other countries, including in the UK, for example, in Tameside, where a *Buurtzorg* model of home care has been contracted since 2016.

- *The Wigan Deal* has seen Wigan Council embark on a major process of change since 2011, involving moving towards asset-based working at scale, empowering communities through a 'citizen-led' approach to public health and creating a culture that permits staff to redesign how they work in response to the needs of individuals and communities. The Wigan Deal is an attempt to strike a new relationship between public services and local people based on four major components: asset-based working; permission to innovate; investing in communities; and place-based neighbourhood working (Naylor and Wellings, 2019).

Developments such as these do raise the issue of how success can be measured. While many organisations have key performance indicators that focus on things that are relatively easy to measure, co-production poses more complex issues. One tool developed by Birmingham University (2019) seeks to develop measures of well-being that are considered to be important to adults. These comprise: *attachment* (an ability to have love, friendship and support); *stability* (an ability to feel settled and secure); *achievement* (an ability to achieve and progress in life); *enjoyment* (an ability to experience enjoyment and pleasure); and *autonomy* (an ability to be independent).

The concept of 'local wealth building' is also relevant here, especially at a strategic system-wide level. This is an approach based on the principle that 'places' hold significant financial, physical and social assets of local institutions and people. The key actors will tend to be local 'anchor' institutions (public, social, academic and commercial) and the focus is upon their procurement role in supporting the local supply chain. This involves opening up – and indeed prioritising – markets to local small and medium-sized enterprises rather than looking to national and international chains. These local suppliers will include employee-owned businesses, social enterprises, cooperatives and other forms of community ownership. Brown et al (2019) identify three key features of the approach: spatial immobility (anchors are unlikely to leave a place once they have taken root, and they have strong ties through invested capital, mission and relationships to customers and employees); size (the employers have significant purchasing power); and not-for-profit status. It is an approach that sits within the stakeholder approach but with the potential to move towards a social contract model.

This has implications for the way adult social care is commissioned since the aim is to ensure that any provider involved in the delivery of services should be as locally generative as possible. As noted by the Centre for Local Economic Studies (2020), this could result in a 'progressive public service marketplace', consisting of: in-house delivery, where the service is delivered by the local state; municipal enterprises, such as arm's-length management organisations and mutually owned companies; worker ownership models; community ownership, such as community businesses, social enterprises and community interest companies; and those local private companies able to demonstrate a concern for the wider community, the environment and staff. Some localities in England are already demonstrating achievements along these lines, notably, in Preston, Manchester, Barnsley and elsewhere (Leibowitz and Goodwin, 2018).

In this respect, social care has to be considered as part of a much broader strategic shift in the way decisions are made and resources are allocated. It is part of a broad remit spanning several council departments and other partners – social care itself, planning, transport, housing, economic development, health, education, criminal justice, community safety, training providers and more. Coordination on this scale would require significant investment in capacity, skills and structures – a point already covered in Chapter 6. The Association for Public Service Excellence (2018), for example, calls for a 'governance framework' to be produced by local councils, identifying all organisations that the council interacts with and creating a shared vision of the development of public services across its area. At the same time, a 'governance forum' is proposed, where all of these organisations meet to pursue a coordinated approach and develop long-term planning. This could require legislation such as an extension of the 'duty to cooperate' so that all public service providers have to engage with councils at the earliest possible time when developing policies. More fundamentally, it requires the reinvention of robust local governance.

Developments like this cannot be purely the product of local, bottom-up action. Too often, innovation in adult social care is fighting against the grain of a sterile top-down national culture. Button and Bedford (2019) identify a number of ways national government could help:

- Creating a 'right to own' by giving employees first refusal to buy out care providers at the point of business transition – in residential care, 30 per cent of beds are provided by small businesses with one home. Supporting employee buy-outs could help to counteract the trend towards these homes being bought out by chain companies when they come up for sale.
- Giving local authorities new powers to buy out providers that are either failing or consistently providing poor-quality care.
- Directing resources towards support for cooperative care transitions and business development along the lines of Co-operative Development Scotland and the Welsh Co-operative Centre. This could play a pivotal role in helping people needing support, their families and care workers to set up social care cooperatives and to take ownership of care businesses in transition.
- Improving access to investment with no expectation of quick or high return for the cooperative, mutual and social enterprise sector so that they are able to play a much greater role in the provision of social care and, above all, residential care. This could involve eligibility for additional payments in much the same way that housing benefit

payments are not capped for some supported living accommodation provided by the not-for-profit sector.

- Strengthening the Care Act 2014 by placing a duty on local authorities to promote diverse forms of democratic ownership across domiciliary and residential social care provision. This duty would be part of local authorities' market-shaping role, which already requires them to 'stimulate a diverse range of care and support services' to ensure that 'people and their carers' have choice over how their needs are met, and that they are able to achieve the things that are important to them.

What is clear from all of this is that thinking about the future of adult social care requires locating it within this wider context. While it is distinctive and essential in its own right, adult social care also needs to be considered in terms of the part it plays in strengthening the places in which we all live. For the Local Government Association (2020a: 5), this means 'moving away from thinking about social care in transactional terms and towards a foundation built on human relationships and connections'.

Commissioning personally

The most prominent policy initiative aimed at encouraging 'personal commissioning' is that of 'personal budgets' and, more recently, personal health budgets. As noted earlier, there have been problems of implementation with this approach, including an unresponsive market, an unwelcoming local authority culture and a narrow conflation of 'personalisation' with the allocation of a sum of money. None of this seems to have dented official enthusiasm for the project. Personal health budgets, in particular, received a boost in the *NHS Long-Term Plan* (NHS England, 2019b), with the aim of reaching 2.6 million people by 2023/24 and then to double that again within a decade. To help achieve this, it was said that over a thousand 'social prescribing link workers' would be in place by 2020/21 and 500 people with 'lived experience' will be trained up to become 'system leaders' by 2023/24.

The difficulties with these forms of individual commissioning are ones of execution rather than conception, for there is evidence of widespread support across local government and the adult care sector for the concept of personalised commissioning (National Audit Office, 2016). To make the model fit for purpose will first require the amounts allocated to be sufficient to meet needs, followed by greater investment in a supportive infrastructure. The House of Commons Committee of

Public Accounts (2017) made a number of recommendations aimed primarily at the Department of Health and Social Care, arguing that it should:

- ensure that published good practice for local authorities and providers shows what high-quality and proportionate support looks like, how much it costs, and that it meets the diverse needs of users;
- explain how it is going to test that all users are receiving genuinely personalised services and that users are receiving the form of personal budget that is most appropriate to their individual circumstances;
- improve its knowledge and understanding of the impact of funding reductions on the adult social care sector; and
- put in place a robust regime to monitor the effectiveness of personal health budgets and of integrated health and social care budgets as it rolls them out, applying relevant lessons from the rolling out of adult social care personal budgets.

The complementary report by the National Audit Office (2016) identified the issues that needed to be addressed at a more local level, in particular: engendering a culture of personalised commissioning; better determination of the amount of users' indicative personal budgets; identifying how to meet users' needs from a broad range of community-based activities; and putting in place adequate and timely user support.

A fundamental issue here is to revisit the concept of personalisation and widen it out from the narrow remit of a financial package. These wider considerations were well encapsulated by the now largely forgotten *Putting People First* strategy (Department of Health, 2007), which set out four dimensions:

- individuals having choice and control over their services through personal budgets;
- widely available low-level support to help people avoid a debilitating crisis;
- universal access to the information needed to make new choices and plans; and
- work to build more inclusive and supported communities.

Of these four, two have been virtually eliminated by austerity – widely available low-level support and work to build more inclusive and supported communities. The personal budget/personal health budget model is one that can and does work for some people (Jones et al,

2017) but there are also those who continue to see it as a step towards the further degrading of a collectivist model and a cover for budget cuts (Slasberg et al, 2015).

Boosting the commissioning role

As noted earlier, public sector commissioning is big business – around a third of all public expenditure (not far short of £300 billion) goes on procurement from external suppliers (Pritchard and Lasko-Skinner, 2019). Given the effective privatisation of provision, adult social care is a significant commissioner in its own right. One recent estimate puts the total direct, indirect and induced value of the sector at 2.6 million jobs and £46.2 billion in 2016 (Skills for Care, 2018a). The likelihood of significant new publicly provided care or any revisiting of the purchaser–provider split seems negligible. This means that there will need to be confidence that the services and supports that are commissioned, contracted and provided meet the needs and requirements of those who rely upon them.

In Chapter 3, it was suggested that the skills and capacity to commission, contract and monitor in adult social care have been diminished by years of austerity, and that there seems to be no strategy to harness the commissioning of public services to some strategic direction. Indeed, we still know remarkably little about those who undertake the commissioning of adult social care. There is no widespread professional accreditation associated with commissioning and the basis of recruitment to the role is far from clear, for example, in terms of previous experience in social work or social care, whether in managerial or front-line positions. In addition, adult social care has never had the sort of investment accorded to the NHS through its 'world class commissioning' programme (McCafferty et al, 2012).

Greater measures could be taken to boost the professional status of commissioning in adult social care. Modest steps have already been taken. The Cabinet Office and its partners have developed the Commissioning Academy, which is designed to equip a small group of professionals to tackle the challenges facing public services and commission the right outcomes for communities. The programme is delivered by the Public Sector Transformation Academy, a not-for-profit social enterprise. It is open to all public sector commissioning organisations, including central government departments, local authorities, health bodies and justice organisations. In the more specific case of adult social care, Skills for Care offers a certificate in Principles of

Commissioning and Wellbeing. Much more of this is needed, probably on a compulsory basis. Elsewhere, localities are taking matters into their own hands, for example, the Greater Manchester Local Commissioning Academy aims to build the capabilities and confidence of public service managers working in commissioning roles.

This needs to be backed up by proper inspection and regulation of the commissioning role. Currently, the adult social care regulator – the Care Quality Commission – has no power to inspect or regulate commissioning. It is common to argue that the strategic role of commissioning and procurement needs to be aligned with strategic policy direction, rather than simply drawing up a menu of 'cost-effective' services. However, this assumes that there is some agreement on the *purpose* of adult social care – an assumption that has been repeatedly questioned throughout this book.

An alternative to the 'market paradigm' for public services has been developed by Lent and Studdert (2019), with their concept of 'the community paradigm'. They see this as underpinned by three broad principles:

- *empowering communities* – shifting decision-making power out of public service institutions into communities, for example, by making more use of social enterprises and community businesses;
- *resourcing communities* – the transfer of core strategic budgets, not just minor discretionary spend; and
- *creating a culture of community collaboration* – breaking the hold of hierarchical and transactional mindsets and developing a more collaborative set of behavioural norms.

These ideas would represent a truly momentous shift in the way service delivery and support is construed and delivered – a seismic shift in commissioning perspective. The way in which Knight et al (2017) depict this is outlined in Table 4.

Chapter summary

This chapter has outlined some components of an 'ethical model' of commissioning in adult social care. It is one that could coexist with a market model, a state model or a combination of both. It is rooted in the importance – indeed, the inescapability – of an ethical foundation for behaviour. In broad terms, it proposes moving away from a 'stockholder' mode through to a 'stakeholder' mode and, more ambitiously, to a 'social contract' mode.

Table 4: Traditional versus new commissioning approaches

Traditional commissioning	New commissioning
Specified scope and outcomes at the outset	Treat scope and outcomes as emergent
Approach implementation as a pilot or project where a model is conceived, tested and evaluated	Favour action-learning over implementation, where viable operating models are an outcome of continuous experimentation
Measure success against predetermined goals	Develop new measures and learning mechanisms as goals and focus emerge and evolve
Aim to produce generalisable findings and models that can be scaled and spread	Produce context-specific understandings about what has worked here, and why, in order to inform ongoing innovation
Maintain a safe distance to ensure independence and objectivity	Work with citizens, communities and providers as an integral part of the process of discovery and learning
Act as the arbiter of what matters, assuming authority over evaluation and judgements of success or failure	Act as the guardian of shared principles and values, engaging with all stakeholders to enable learning and understanding

Source: Knight et al (2017)

In all of this, it is assumed that those working in adult social care are – or certainly should be – active moral agents, guided by ethical principles and making a critical interpretation of relevant ethical codes. However, this goes beyond individual practitioners. Public policies are about what governments choose to do (or choose not to do) and what principles should guide their decision-making. In this sense, ethics lies at the heart of public policy and all aspects of the policymaking cycle.

Four suggestions are made for incorporating an ethical focus into adult social care commissioning (and hence provision): commissioning ethical employment practice; commissioning for well-being; commissioning local and small; and commissioning personally. There is evidence that each of them is currently in use but that they tend to be confined to a handful of progressive localities or exist nationally in only nascent form. It is suggested that a combination of support and regulation could help to make a difference.

8

COVID-19: the stress test of adult social care

Introduction

This is a chapter that was not envisaged when the proposal for this book was submitted in 2019. Much has happened since then, and continues to evolve; therefore, this chapter can still be little more than an early commentary on the impact of COVID-19 on the adult social care 'system'. What is clear, however, is that COVID-19 thrust adult social care into public awareness and political consciousness in an unexpected and startling way, the longer-term consequences of which remain uncertain (Department of Health and Social Care, 2020f).

The narrative throughout this volume has been of a model of commissioning and provision that has been struggling, if not failing outright, and that could therefore easily be destabilised by any of its inherent weaknesses. Prior to 2020, the forces of destabilisation tended to be around funding shortfalls and a fragile provider market. COVID-19 constituted something very different: a colossal stress test of everything previously taken for granted about the economic, political and social order. The timing of the virus was unanticipated, the severity underestimated and the preparedness barely existent; adult social care was soon caught in its headlights.

The immediate response was around clinical matters – testing, tracing and tracking, the acquisition of personal protective equipment (PPE), and the curtailment of business activity and social interactions via lockdown. However, the pandemic also created some very specific challenges for adult social care and, in so doing, revealed much about the way the sector is perceived by politicians and policymakers. These challenges reflect many of the issues analysed in the preceding chapters, notably:

- deficiencies in funding and administration
- fragility of provision
- low policy salience
- unethical policy and practice

Deficiencies in funding and administration

Chapter 6 drew attention to the ad hoc 'sticking plaster' model of funding for local government and, by extension, adult social care – a confusing mix of modest sums to fix crisis-related problems, often distributed through NHS organisations and unrelated to any coherent strategy for the sector. The COVID-19 crisis witnessed a continuation of this approach; within the space of three months, no less than eight new pots of money were allocated from central government to ameliorate the impact of the pandemic on local government.

Vital municipal income streams soon began to dry up once the country had gone into lockdown – early estimates were of more than £400 million lost in business rates, £288 million in council tax losses and £341 million in fees and charges. To help counteract this, local authorities received two chunks of new funding from central government. An initial allocation of £1.6 billion was made available to help manage pressures across all council services, one of which would clearly be adult social care. Here, the money was expected to be used to: protect providers' cash flows; monitor the ongoing costs of delivering care (such as higher workforce absence rates caused by self-isolation and the cost of buying PPE); and adjust fees to meet new costs. A further tranche of £1.3 billion was specifically intended to rapidly free up 15,000 hospital beds for COVID-19 patients by expediting discharge from hospital back home or to alternative accommodation (notably, care homes) for those patients for whom a clinical setting was no longer deemed appropriate. The government also paid upfront £850 million of social care grant that would otherwise have been paid monthly and allowed councils to defer payments to central government of £2.5 billion in business rates. The latter two interventions obviously required repayment further down the line (Institute for Fiscal Studies, 2020).

These amounts were soon a matter of dispute, both over their size and distribution. Disagreement arose between councils and care providers over the amounts allocated to cover increasing care costs: the 5 per cent uplift to cover the National Living Wage uplift was said to be insufficient to cover the true rise of 6.25 per cent; and the 10 per cent increase generally awarded for additional costs associated with COVID-19 was said to be insufficient to even cover the increased costs of purchasing PPE and related workforce costs. The allocation also led to dispute within the local government sector between those councils with social care responsibilities and district councils that hold responsibility for other vital services – the latter took the view that their needs were being ignored.

This fragile funding base soon led the Association of Directors of Adult Social Services to take the unusual step of lodging a complaint with the Director General of Community and Social Care at the Department of Health and Social Care about the imbalance between central government understandings of the requirements of the NHS as opposed to those of adult social care. Councils had intervened as best they could with resources they did not possess, providing PPE to care workers, housing rough sleepers, attempting to improve mental health support and protecting people at risk of domestic abuse. There was thought to be an understanding between central and local government that councils should do 'whatever it took' to respond to local need, with an assurance that the additional costs would be met. Councils subsequently discovered this not to be the case.

Unlike the NHS, local government has no room for fiscal manoeuvre. Not only are their own revenue-raising powers very limited, but they are also legally required to balance annual budgets. In the wake of extra spending on COVID-19, some councils were said to be at risk of formal bankruptcy notifications within weeks. In response, a further £1 billion was found by central government, a sum dismissed by councils as only sufficient to cover increased costs for a month or two. Again, in response to fresh concerns about the high death rate in care homes, a new £600 million Infection Control Fund was created. This only added further to the confusing mix of income streams, this time also with demanding reporting requirements on the precise use of the allocation in a manner more suited to dealing with a contractor than with a democratically elected tier of governance. Overall, although unprecedented sums had rapidly been found to buttress businesses and employees during the lockdown, there was no real change to the 'sticking plaster' regime for local government (Department of Health and Social Care, 2020g).

These problems with the funding of local government arise directly from the organisational weakness of the sector itself – an issue also explored in Chapter 6. The arrival of COVID-19 suddenly pushed the state and the public sector into the forefront of intervention; however, by then, the local and regional infrastructure of the state had been badly damaged in the period between 2010 and 2020, when these tiers were stripped of experience and capacity. Although responses to the pandemic required granular localised responses, local authorities were again marginalised by central government.

The default preference for outsourcing to the private sector is the other side of the coin to this destruction of municipalism. As old structures of governance were eviscerated, the gap was filled by private companies whose expertise lay in bidding for large contracts and offering immediate delivery. Testing for the virus was outsourced to private companies, as was the distribution of emergency food vouchers; the tracing and tracking of the infection was centralised within Public Health England, leaving around 5,000 environmental health officers (employed by local councils) unused; and the contract for a subsequent nationwide tracing and tracking programme was also handed over to the private sector. By the middle of May 2020, it was estimated that £1.7 billion of state contracts (usually without tender) had been awarded to private companies and around £125 billion had been committed by government to a range of programmes and initiatives (National Audit Office, 2020a).

Fragility of provision

Fragility in the care market

Concerns about the way that organisations providing care and support receive and use their funding have been a recurring theme of this volume. The COVID-19 pandemic intensified these concerns (ADASS, 2020). Chapter 4 explored the diversity and fragmentation of the sector, with thousands of independent companies making their own decisions on where to set up, what to provide and whether or not to continue. The fact that these companies exist as separate businesses in competition with one another has made it more difficult for them to collaborate to jointly procure protective equipment, or reallocate staff members from one home to another to cover sickness absences. It has also made the sector much less susceptible to the command-and-control diktats from government that have been applied to the NHS.

The casualised nature of the workforce (also examined in Chapter 4) created further difficulties in trying to cope with COVID-19. Care workers were sometimes working in more than one care setting – providing care services in someone's home one day, while working in a residential care setting the next – thus potentially increasing the spread of the disease among those most vulnerable. Agency staff are often employed on zero-hours contracts and make up around 10 per cent of the adult social care workforce. They are a prominent feature of care home settings, where they are three times more likely to be used than in other parts of the labour market (Office for National Statistics, 2020a). Similarly, the reliance on zero-hours contracts in the home care sector heightened the risk that those workers who were sick with the virus would feel unable to afford to stay at home and isolate. One early piece of work on the issue (Hayes et al, 2020) reported that 80 per cent of care workers did not expect to be paid their normal wages if they had to self-isolate due to COVID-19 and were accordingly reluctant to self-isolate. Unlike the NHS, care providers are not legally required to provide occupational sick pay and most do not do so.

The fragile financial structure of the industry meant that most providers were already unable to withstand even a minor downturn in income or an increase in costs. In this respect, COVID-19 was immediately seismic in its impact. Once the virus began to take hold, there were increased costs associated with hygiene, PPE and staff costs, alongside a fall in income and occupancy levels due to the widespread premature deaths of large numbers of older people. Many of the people who died during the pandemic would already have been receiving care and support, or would have been at high risk of needing it in the near future, both of which will impact upon post-pandemic levels of demand. Councils, in turn, will be faced with helping to meet the shortfall through higher fees; otherwise, they will risk losing their local markets. However, in the absence of a huge and sustainable increase in funding, they will be unable to do so.

For both care home providers and home care agencies, these events have provided a serious threat to business viability. With some estimates of over 20,000 deaths in care homes, occupancy rates began to slip towards 80 per cent – a level deemed incompatible with financial survival. Concerns were soon being expressed that the sector was heading towards a financial collapse. The Care Providers Alliance (representing about half of all care providers) was warning that without emergency funding to help pay wages and buy PPE, the sector risked collapse. In addition, the biggest care home provider in the UK – HC-One – noted in its accounts for 2019 that the impact of the pandemic on its occupancy levels and cash flow had cast significant doubt on the group's ability to continue as a going concern. Meanwhile, the UK Home Care Association was warning that the financial pressures arising from COVID-19 could force a significant number of the country's 8,000 home care providers to close within weeks. The fragmentation and fragility of the care market was soon starkly exposed.

Fragility in the voluntary sector

Weaknesses in the third sector were also intensified by COVID-19. The most immediate impact was upon finances, which – as explored in Chapter 4 – were already in a precarious position. Bookings for training and services were cancelled, charity shops closed, community fundraising halted and (in the case of the larger charities) investment portfolios reduced in value. A survey of the sector undertaken during the lockdown period by the Directory of Social Change (2020) revealed some alarming findings:

- half said that they were already in financial difficulties due to the pandemic, with another 42 per cent expecting to be soon;
- over 60 per cent were furloughing staff under the Coronavirus Job Retention Scheme;
- only 7 per cent qualified for help via the Coronavirus Business Interruption Loan Scheme; and
- over half said they would be bankrupt within six months without financial help.

The government could have taken urgent steps to bolster the sector in a number of ways: an emergency grant fund; the deferral of national insurance contributions and VAT payments; a loan guarantee offer for charities needing overdrafts to cover cash flow; the upfront payment of existing grants; flexibility on reporting and monitoring; and freedom to use funding in more flexible ways (Centre for Social Justice, 2020). In the event, the Chancellor announced an injection of £750 million into the sector, of which £360 million would be directly allocated by government departments and £370 million would go to small local charities.

Although seen as a welcome step, this allocation was generally viewed as insufficient by the sector, which – on its own estimation – had lost around £4 billion in the few weeks since the outbreak of the virus. An expeditious inquiry by the Commons Digital, Culture, Media and Sports Committee (2020) found charities to be fighting for survival, with smaller charities at risk of imminent closure. The £750 million support was denounced by the committee as insufficient, lacking transparency in its allocation and unduly prioritising those organisations directly assisting health and social care services on the front line of tackling COVID-19. It went on to call on the government to increase the support available through a comprehensive stabilisation fund and to make this more widely available to charities doing essential work that was not directly focused on COVID-19. In the face of this criticism, a further tranche of £150 million was created (mostly by accessing dormant bank accounts) to expand emergency loans to charities. As with local government funding, it is a crisis-driven 'sticking plaster' model of support.

One of the most interesting social effects of the pandemic was the spontaneous flowering of many (largely unrecorded) local and neighbourhood self-help groups (Tiratelli and Kaye, 2020). These are likely to have numbered several thousands, typically making use of WhatsApp communication and other means to support people needing help with shopping and picking up prescriptions, or requiring moral support. The All–Party Parliamentary Group on Social Integration (2020) estimated that by the end of March 2020, around 300,000 people had volunteered with local organisations in this way. These groups were largely ignored by official responses; instead, the government sought to develop a completely new model of support, developed and administered centrally, that of the 'NHS Volunteer' scheme. This aimed to recruit around 750,000 volunteers in England to help the NHS support the estimated 1.5 million people with complex health needs who had been designated as 'shielded' and thereby required to stay at home in all circumstances for at least three months.

Although dubbed 'NHS Volunteers', the tasks required to be undertaken more resembled the functions of adult social care. Four roles were identified:

- *community response volunteers*, who would collect shopping, medication or other essential supplies for someone self-isolating and deliver these to their home;
- *patient transport volunteers*, who would drive discharged patients back to their homes or other accommodation;
- *NHS transport volunteers*, who would move equipment, supplies or medication between sites; and
- *check-in and chat volunteers*, who would provide regular support calls to elderly people living in isolation and at risk of loneliness.

The first and last of these roles involve no engagement with the NHS at all, and could certainly have been expected to overlap or clash with the efforts of neighbourhood groups and established local charities. The government preferred a centralised model, drawing upon new technologies. Those recruited as volunteers were directed to use an app through which they could say they were 'on duty'. GPs, doctors, pharmacists, nurses, midwives, NHS 111 advisers and social care staff were all then able to request help via a national call centre run by the Royal Voluntary Service, which was expected to match volunteers with people living near to them who needed help.

This was clearly a massive logistical exercise that might have been better administered by local councils rather than from a centralised telephone line, especially with a view to sustaining these networks of support beyond the duration of the crisis. Volunteering (other than in the acute hospital setting) has never been central to the way the NHS is run and the fact that the government preferred this NHS-oriented top-down model rather than asking local councils and voluntary groups to coordinate efforts is telling. Evaluations of the impact of this scheme may emerge in due course but early reports suggest considerable difficulty in matching the availability of volunteers to local needs.

Overall, the impact of COVID-19 on the voluntary sector has been paradoxical. On the one hand, much of the sector has been pushed to the point of financial ruin. On the other hand, many more people turned to volunteering than would have otherwise been the case – some estimates suggested up to 10 million people had 'volunteered' in some way (Legal & General, 2020). If this level of contribution can survive into the longer term, there could be the potential to increase levels of social connection, reciprocity and trust (Office for National Statistics, 2020b).

Low policy salience

A recurring theme in this volume has been the low policy salience accorded to what is now commonly termed 'adult social care'. From the Victorian Poor Law onwards, it has struggled to be seen as anything other than a residual means-tested service, and it has accordingly received relatively little political attention. Notwithstanding official requests to 'clap for carers' and the invention of a new 'carers badge', this situation was not in any way rectified in the wake of COVID-19. Indeed, if anything, it was exacerbated in two significant ways: the easement of statutory duties; and the perception of the sector as a handmaiden to the needs of the NHS.

Easement of statutory duties

Rather than ensure that local councils were adequately funded and empowered to respond to the challenges thrown up by COVID-19, one of the first responses of the government was to relieve them of their existing statutory obligations. The Coronavirus Act 2020 provided for the 'easement' of local authority duties in England and Wales relating to the provision of care and support needs. This meant that they would no longer have to comply with their duty under the Care Act 2014 to conduct needs assessments and provide support, unless failing to do so might constitute a breach of a person's human rights. The latter constituted a very high bar indeed.

The accompanying impact assessment stated that without these legislative relaxations, local authorities would be unduly constrained by existing assessments, which might then be maintained at the expense of new and more urgent needs (House of Commons Library, 2020c). Indeed, during the second reading of the Coronavirus Bill, the Health Secretary seemed to raise the bar for access to support even higher – to a matter of life and death. He stated that:

> The purpose of these measures is to make sure that when there is a shortage of social care workers, those who need social care to live their everyday life get it and can be prioritised ahead of those who have a current legal right to social care under the Care Act 2014, but for whom it is not a matter of life and death.

Given the very tight criteria for access to support that pertained prior to the virus crisis (see Chapter 4), it is clear that individuals with very substantial needs could no longer expect to have access to support. Guidance from the Department of Health and Social Care (2020c) went on to identify four key areas where the obligations of the Care Act 2014 could be changed, with local authorities no longer having to: carry out detailed assessments of people's care and support needs; carry out financial assessments (though charges can be applied retrospectively); prepare or review care and support plans; and meet eligible care and support needs.

These statutory relaxations are part of the vast legislation contained within the Coronavirus Act 2020, which runs to 328 pages and has a further 73 pages of explanatory notes. The relaxations are intended to be time-limited to two years, though a minister may extend the provisions for a further six months at a time. Given the poor understanding of the nature of the virus and the length of time needed to develop and make available an effective vaccine, these measures could stay in place for a prolonged period.

Within weeks of availability, eight areas had taken up powers of easement even though there was emerging evidence of a *decline* in the number of people coming forward to seek help – a phenomenon fuelled by a combination of fear of contracting the virus, alongside the fresh support coming from the newly created neighbourhood groups (Bolton, 2020). This soon led to allegations that the measures had been adopted without the necessary legal justification. The guidance accompanying the powers stated that a local authority should only take a decision to proceed when the workforce was significantly depleted or demand had increased to the point where compliance with the Care Act 2014 would potentially risk life. Concerns were expressed that local authorities were entering into easement without providing evidence of meeting these thresholds. In some cases, legal action was taken and this led initially to a reduction in the number of councils using these new powers.

Various other forms of relaxation were also introduced in the Act. One related to the use of NHS 'continuing health care' (CHC) assessments. Clause 13 of the Act allows NHS providers to delay undertaking the assessment process for CHCs until after the pandemic has ended. The view of the government was that this would enable patients to be discharged from hospital more quickly in order to free up hospital space; it also meant that the individuals involved would then be means-tested for their alternative social care provision. The threshold for social work registration by Social Work England was also lowered and routine inspections by the Care Quality Commission were suspended.

The relaxation of inspections by the regulator during the pandemic is surprising. As Hayes et al (2020) note, the legal function of inspection is to establish whether the provision of care meets basic standards of safety and quality. These are set out in law and cover matters such as sufficient staff numbers, safe care practices and the provision of adequate food and hydration. Without routine inspection, there was no mechanism for systematic examination of the care being provided during the pandemic, or of the impact of COVID-19 in care settings. The Health and Social Care Act 2012 had already removed the power of the Health and Safety Executive to perform spot checks on social care establishments.

Overall, in England, the legislative response to COVID-19 was to relieve local authorities of their obligations to assess and provide support, and to reduce requirements on regulatory bodies to inspect services. A somewhat different position was taken in Scotland, where the Coronavirus (Scotland) (No.2) Act 2020 included provisions giving local authorities and health boards new powers to take over the running of care homes and even to acquire businesses and assets themselves where the provider is in serious financial difficulty or there is a threat to the health and well-being of the persons receiving services.

Adult social care and the NHS

Reference was made in Chapter 6 to the tangled relationship between adult social care and the NHS, amid concerns that the shape of the former was increasingly being determined by the needs of the latter. These concerns were amplified in the wake of the pandemic, when the focus from the outset was on the NHS, as exemplified in the slogan 'Protect the

NHS' and the constant political injunction to ensure that the NHS was not overwhelmed. The two sectors were treated very differently in terms of the availability of funding, testing and PPE, and even in the ways deaths were counted (Commons Public Accounts Committee 2020a; 2020b).

The spread of COVID-19 was always bound to be substantially different in residential settings than in the general population since residents are usually older adults who have multiple illnesses, functional impairment, dementia and high mortality if they contract the disease. Physical distancing is not possible for most residents because of their frailty and close living quarters, and the quarantining of symptomatic residents is not always possible. The failure to foresee the importance of testing kit and PPE in care home environments was a serious mistake that cost many lives. Hayes et al (2020) found a large majority of care and support workers saying that their employers were not doing enough to keep them or the people they worked with safe from infection. The researchers concluded that there was considerable confusion in guidance issued by the Department of Health about whether, when and why PPE was necessary in care settings.

These errors soon led to rocketing numbers of deaths in care settings, especially care homes. While COVID-19-related hospital deaths were reported on a daily basis, those in other settings were reported only weekly until political pressure resolved the variation. The Care Quality Commission belatedly began to record the number of COVID-19 deaths in care homes but it was unclear how this could be done with accuracy given the low rate of testing. Towards the end of April 2020, it was estimated that almost 11,000 more people than normal had died in care homes since the start of the outbreak, compared with the official estimate of 1,034. This was in line with international data which suggested that care home residents were accounting for between 42 per cent and 57 per cent of all deaths related to COVID-19 (International Long-term Care Policy Network, 2020). Figures on deaths from COVID-19 among adults with learning disabilities were harder to trace but the rates were eventually found to be more than double those of previous years. Even these figures excluded those detained in hospital or subject to community measures under the Mental Health Act 1983.

The subsequent *Action Plan* published by the Department of Health and Social Care (2020a) stated that 'the government's "number one priority" for adult social care was for everyone who relies on care to get the care they need throughout the COVID-19 pandemic'. The strategy was said to rest on four pillars: controlling the spread of infection; supporting the workforce; supporting independence, supporting people at the end of their lives and responding to individual needs; and supporting local authorities and the providers of care. The plan failed to bolster confidence within the sector, nor did a reprise of the oft-repeated line that the government would bring forward a plan for social care for the longer term (Department of Health and Social Care, 2020e). The value of the Social Care Sector COVID-19 Support Task Force (belatedly created to oversee the delivery of the *Action Plan*) remains to be seen (Department of Health and Social Care, 2020d).

Unethical policy and practice

The ethical framework for adult social care

Chapter 7 explored the relative absence of ethical reflection and its place in policy and practice in adult social care. It took the COVID-19 outbreak to finally produce an 'ethical framework' for the sector (Department of Health and Social Care, 2020b). The framework aimed 'to ensure that ample consideration be given to a series of ethical values and principles when organising and delivering care for adults' (Department of Health and Social Care, 2020b: 3). Eight principles were identified:

- *respect* – recognising that every person and their human rights, personal choices, safety and dignity matters;
- *reasonableness* – ensuring that decisions are rational, fair, practical and grounded in appropriate processes, available evidence and a clear justification;
- *minimising harm* – striving to reduce the amount of physical, psychological, social and economic harm that the outbreak might cause to individuals and communities;
- *inclusiveness* – ensuring people are given a fair opportunity to understand individual situations, be included in decisions that affect them and offer their views and challenge;
- *accountability* – holding people, and ourselves, to account for how and which decisions are made, as well as being transparent about why decisions are made and who is responsible for making and communicating them;
- *flexibility* – being responsive, able and willing to adapt when faced with changed or new circumstances;
- *proportionality* – providing support that is proportional to needs and abilities of people, communities and the staff; and
- *community* – a commitment to get through the outbreak together by supporting one another and strengthening our communities to the best of our ability.

These are useful principles to guide behaviour in any circumstances and it might be considered unfortunate that it took a global pandemic for them to be formulated. Guidance from the government set out 'an expectation' that local authorities would 'observe' the framework. Indeed, it went further, stating that alongside the framework, local authorities should 'continue to respect the principles of personalisation and coproduction' (Department of Health and Social Care, 2020b). The application of the ethical principles in the face of tightening of access to support is bound to be fraught – if not impossible – to deliver. Indeed, in a classic understatement, it was acknowledged within the framework that the implementation of these values and principles could 'encounter tension between them which will require a judgement to be made on the extent that a particular value or principle can be applied in the context of each particular decision' (Department of Health and Social Care, 2020b: 4).

COVID-19 and age discrimination

The ethical framework might be considered to be at odds with some of the ageist policy overtures associated with the political and scientific interest in 'herd immunity' – an epidemiological concept that describes the state whereby a population is sufficiently immune to a disease such that the infection will not spread to more vulnerable people. In the early stage of the response to the virus, this was presented as a preventive strategy that could stall the spread of disease. It was central to the government's decision-making in the crucial months of February and March but, crucially, there was no parallel strategy to protect the most vulnerable. This situation was only abandoned when it became clear that the NHS would be overwhelmed and hundreds of thousands of citizens could die – up to 250,000 deaths, mostly of older people, were predicted in an advice paper from Imperial College London (Propper et al., 2020).

The implied acceptance of the deaths of large numbers of older and more vulnerable people was also evident in other policies. As noted earlier, local councils were awarded £2.9 billion from the Treasury's COVID-19 fund, of which £1.3 billion was intended to 'enhance' hospital discharge in order to free up 15,000 beds for COVID-19 patients. The 'easement' of the requirements around CHCs represented a further attempt to clear beds more quickly than normal. It soon became clear that the care home sector in particular was a breeding ground for infection and death from COVID-19. This situation arose partly from the lack of protective equipment for residents and staff but also from the failure of NHS trusts to test discharged patients for the virus prior to transfer from hospitals to care homes (National Audit Office, 2020b). The advice in government guidance that such admissions would be safe as long as social distancing rules were applied soon turned out to be impractical and deadly.

Reports also emerged of residents in some care homes for older people (and adults with learning disability) being categorised en masse as not requiring resuscitation should they contract the disease (Office for National Statistics, 2020c). The Care Quality Commission had to step in and issue a warning for the practice to stop. It was as if the deaths from COVID-19 of people over 70 and those with 'underlying health conditions' was the natural order of things. A similar tale applied to adults of working age, with the National Institute for Health and Clinical Excellence (NICE) forced to change its advice to the NHS to deny disabled people treatment after disability groups threatened legal action. NICE had told doctors that they should assess patients with conditions such as learning disability and autism as scoring high for 'frailty' (thereby meeting the criteria to be refused treatment) based on the fact that they needed support with personal care in their day-to-day lives. This reflects the wider 'demonisation' of disabled people described more fully by Ryan (2019).

There is an important strand of highly unethical behaviour associated with these events. The assumption behind 'herd immunity' was that the pandemic could be contained if it was allowed to spread largely unhindered in the wider community. However, the quid pro quo for this would have to be that vulnerable people are protected, especially those living in residential settings. This implied the need for careful government monitoring, the efficient supply of PPE, the widespread availability of testing and reduced exposure to visitors and other carers. None of these were assured and the sector was left to cope on its own at great human cost for too long. Reports emerged, for example, of councils refusing to use their COVID-19 funding streams to support care homes *unless* they agreed to take in COVID-19-confirmed patients. This will also have contributed directly to subsequent findings that the rate of COVID-19 deaths among social care staff far outstripped those of healthcare workers and the wider working population.

It is also difficult to avoid the conclusion that all of this was foreseeable and, to some extent, preventable. In 2016, Public Health England ran Exercise Cygnus to assess preparedness for a pandemic. This involved coordinating the contributions of almost a thousand people from central government, teams of local emergency planners, prison officers and others to test the UK's capacity to respond to a new global pandemic.

The report has never been published, but is thought to have concluded that plans, policies and capability were all insufficient. One of its recommendations included boosting the capacity of care homes and the numbers of staff available to work in them, while also warning of the dangers of asking care homes to take in patients discharged from hospital. Ethical considerations apply as much to policy omissions as to policy actions.

Revaluing the workforce

Chapter 4 examined the low valuation that has been put upon the adult social care workforce, as reflected in low pay, job insecurity, inadequate training and low status. The dedication and sacrifices of care staff in the face of COVID-19 led to a wider understanding and appreciation of their role, and resulted in talk of a new 'moral economy' – a reappraisal of which jobs are most important in a modern economy. Thomas and Quilter-Pinner (2020), for example, called for five 'core guarantees' to the health and care workforce: a safety guarantee; an accommodation guarantee; a mental health guarantee; a pay guarantee (10 per cent pay bonus); and a care guarantee (funding childcare provision). In the event, the only immediate response in the government's *Action Plan* in the case of care staff was the designation of a badge for care workers to expedite their access to supermarket shopping. The longer-term consequences of the pandemic on the workforce remain unclear.

There is no clarity on the future of the sector in the wake of the pandemic. The wider recognition of the role it plays in society could easily be lost in a post-pandemic economic crisis where a government traditionally wedded to a small-state, low-tax model of government will be faced with a challenging environment. By May 2020, attempts to cushion the economic fallout arising from COVID-19 were reckoned to be creating a budget deficit of around £440 billion, as compared with a deficit of £55 billion before the pandemic struck. This deficit could be tackled in four ways: a return to austerity, tax rises, encouraging economic growth and higher borrowing. It would be optimistic to think that in these circumstances, there will be any significant investment in public services in general or adult social care in particular.

Chapter summary

All told, the role of the adult social care sector in responding to the COVID-19 crisis has tended to reflect its policy marginality. The rapidly released funding was a continuation of the 'sticking plaster' approach that has characterised government responses for the last decade. The emergency legislation rapidly rewrote and downgraded the legal obligations of councils to assess need and respond to those eligible for support. The efforts to hugely harness the role of volunteers was determined centrally and delivered via a top-down model. The focus on releasing hospital beds reinforced the perception of adult social care as a second-class auxiliary health service. Finally, the underpinning assumption seemed to imply that the lives of those likely to need care services and support were of secondary value to the need for economic recovery.

The pandemic certainly demonstrated that, when necessary, the state can act in transformative ways, both in terms of massive state funding and ambitious strategies that challenge the status quo, but none of this seemed to apply to adult social care. The government's *Action Plan* was seemingly based upon the assumption that the social care system could be sorted out by building on an existing dysfunctional market structure. The danger was that once the pandemic subsided, the prospects for a meaningful debate about the nature, purpose and structure of the sector would, once again, be lost.

9

Conclusion: making it change – morals, markets and power

Introduction

As Chapter 8 noted, the advent of COVID-19 resulted in the creation of an official ethical framework for adult social care. However, even where ethical ideals are pronounced by government or expressed in organisational mission statements, it is unlikely that they will be much discussed in practice and turned into realistic measures to guide action. Indeed, the most common discussions about ethics tend to be of *breaches* of integrity, such as intimidation, discrimination, manipulation of information, breaking rules and conflicts of interest (Huberts, 2018). It is therefore important to be clear not only about what is understood by new ethical standards (see Chapters 7 and 8), but also how ethical behaviour can be more robustly incorporated into the way services (and indeed goods) can be delivered.

Instilling ethical behaviour

In England, the most notable attempt to address the place of ethics in public life was the creation of the Committee on Standards in Public Life (CSPL) by the then Prime Minister John Major in 1994. The task of the CSPL was 'to examine current concerns about standards of conduct of all holders of public office, including arrangements relating to financial and commercial activities'. The CSPL went on to articulate seven principles of public life, now often referred to as the 'Nolan Principles': selflessness, integrity, objectivity, accountability, openness, honesty and leadership (Bew, 2015).

In 2014, the CSPL published a review of the application of these standards to the provision of public services (Committee on Standards in Public Life, 2014) and formed several conclusions: that the public wanted common ethical standards regardless of sector, supported by a code of conduct; that 'how' the service is delivered is as important to the public as 'what' is delivered, with a wish for personalisation and a user-led definition of quality; that public and stakeholder views of what should constitute ethical standards were broadly in line with the Nolan Principles; that commissioners expect providers to conform to ethical standards but rarely explicitly articulate this; and that commissioners themselves wanted guidance on how to embed ethical standards in the commissioning and procurement process. All of this is highly relevant to an ethical basis for the commissioning and delivery of adult social care. Three recommendations were made in a subsequent CSPL report in 2018 (Committee on Standards in Public Life, 2018):

- that all public service providers must, at the point of commissioning, agree to the commissioning body's statement of intent on the ethical behaviour expected of the board, employees and subcontractors in the delivery of any contract;
- that all public service providers must, at the point of commissioning, publish a corollary 'statement of provider's intent', showing their plan for embedding a culture of high ethical standards in their service delivery; and
- that those managing contracts need additional ethical training in relation to service delivery – principles and codes of practice are insufficient.

There is little evidence to suggest that these recommendations have been widely observed in adult social care or, indeed, elsewhere in the public sector. In response to the collapse of Carillion in 2018, the government published its *Outsourcing Playbook* (Government Commercial Function, 2019), outlining guidance on the way outsourcing should be undertaken. A review a year later (Sasse et al, 2020) could find little evidence of improvements to the way government assesses risk and balances cost and quality, or of awareness of the existence of the guidance in local government and other public bodies, including the NHS.

Further measures are clearly needed. The first is ethical leadership – a clear message from the top of an organisation that ethical behaviour really matters. One useful example from the field of education is the Ethical Leadership Commission (Association of School and College Leaders, 2019) founded by head teachers. This group was tasked with creating a set of values to help school leaders navigate an educational 'moral maze' in which a preoccupation with results had led to such incidents as 'off-rolling', exam cheating and channelling students into easier subjects. The commission took as its starting point the Nolan Principles but then added a number of other characteristics of good leadership: trust, wisdom, kindness, justice, service, courage and optimism. By 2020, over a hundred schools were trialling the framework in relation to real-life dilemmas. Something similar is needed for adult social care and, indeed, other public services domains, along with the opportunity to join up at the national level. However, it is not just about leadership; managers and front-line practitioners also need time and space to develop and apply ethical competence, rather than having to endlessly cope with day-to-day crisis interventions.

Second, at a broader level, there are lessons to be learned from other countries. Respect for evidence in policy design is crucial, but despite much political rhetoric about 'evidence-based policy', too many policies are flawed in design and fail to address the problems they were set up to address (Hudson et al, 2019). As noted in Chapter 2, in the case of adult social care, the introduction of a market model was an evidence-free shift based upon a leap of ideological faith. This deficiency was then compounded by inadequate use of data in monitoring policy implementation. In the US, the Commission on Evidence-Based Policymaking set up in 2016 issued its final report 18 months later (Commission on Evidence-Based Policymaking, 2017), which outlined a vision for 'a future in which rigorous evidence is created efficiently as a routine part of government operations and used to construct effective public policy'. These recommendations subsequently became federal law in the Foundations for Evidence-Based Policymaking Act. It is unclear, however, how well this model has been able to operate in the face of the Trump presidency.

Finally, there is the need for some form of institutional check on breaches of integrity. As currently constituted, the CSPL lacks the powers to undertake such a role but a stronger model is observable in Australia, where the 2018 National Integrity Commission Bill sought to establish an Australian National Integrity Commission as an independent public sector anti-corruption commission. Although there are ongoing criticisms of the likely limitations of the remit that such a commission might cover, it is nevertheless an important debate that is yet to even start in the UK.

Morals and markets

Chapter 5 explored some of the issues around the 'state versus market' argument in relation to adult social care and Chapter 7 articulated the contours of an ethical model for the sector. When the logic of buying and selling no longer applies to material goods alone, but also to sensitive domains like adult social care, questions will inevitably arise about the appropriateness of the penetration of market values. The philosopher Michael Sandel (2012) argues that markets have become detached from morals and have expanded into spheres of life where they do not belong, leading to non-market values having been crowded out in the process. In effect, and with little debate, the UK has drifted from *having* a market economy to *being* a market society.

The danger is that this can lead to a decline in the ethical values that are normally associated with notions of 'care'. In her analysis of the loss of kindness in public policy, Unwin (2018) identifies two lexicons. First, there is the language of metrics and value added, of growth and resource allocation, of regulation, and of impact. On the other hand, there is the language of kindness and grief, of loneliness, love and friendship, and of the ties that bind and our sense of identity and belonging. Both vocabularies, she says, have strengths but each is inadequate on its own. The concern is that the first language has dominated over recent decades. The public choice school theorists (Buchanan and Tullock, 1962) simply *asserted* that politicians, bureaucrats and their voters were self-interested economic actors like any others in a marketplace: people who made calculations of the costs and benefits of their actions on the back of perfect information about their options. In fact, as seen in the case of those purchasing their own care and support, the greater the complexity of a good or product, the higher the risk of 'asymmetrical' contracts in which the seller has more information than the buyer and hence can exploit that buyer.

On the back of public choice theory was the rise in popularity of 'new public management' (Hood, 1991), whereby many public services were outsourced to the commercial sector and cost became the key proxy for value. Arguably, adult social care became the exemplar of this approach. The contrary position is that public services are based upon the notion of a unique set of public values, distinct from the personal or commercial, representing the common good, democracy, public interest and social cohesion. The erosion of this position has commercialised the relationship between the local/national state and citizens, which is now often indistinguishable from that of producer and consumer. As a consequence, the democratic nature of public services has been severely undermined and citizens are viewed not as people with rights to public goods, but as consumers of services bought by them or procured on their behalf (Centre for Local Economic Studies, 2020).

Some 50 years ago, Richard Titmuss (1997 [1970]), in *The Gift Relationship*, argued in favour of the UK system of voluntary blood donation and against treating human blood as a commodity to be bought and sold on the market. He further argued that the latter not only eroded people's sense of obligation to donate blood, but also diminished the spirit of altruism and undermined the 'gift relationship'. This relates to Sandel's claim that the danger now is that in an era of market triumphalism, public discourse is drained of moral and civic energy. To decide where the market belongs, and where it should be kept at a distance, decisions have to be explicitly made about how to value the goods and services in question – adult social care, health, education, family life and so on. These are moral and political questions, not merely economic ones.

Policy failure in adult social care

Most policies end up failing in some degree but a common thread throughout this book is that adult social care has relatively few successes to its credit. As McConnell (2015) has noted, 'failure' resides at the extreme end of a success–failure spectrum, where it is characterised by absolute non-achievement. Such a situation will be unusual. He observes that 'failure is rarely unequivocal and absolute ... even policies that have become known as classic policy failures also produced small and modest successes' (McConnell, 2015: 231). It would be churlish to claim that adult social care has been devoid of some success but – as evidenced in Chapters 3 and 4 – the market era has ended up largely in a state of failure.

An influential review of failure in major government projects in the UK by the National Audit Office (2013) identified five interacting factors that often contributed to 'over-optimism' in policymaking:

- *Complexity*: public bodies too often underestimate the delivery challenges of complex projects and fail to spend time to deepen their understanding. There is a commitment to a 'solution' with insufficient understanding of the context and options.
- *Evidence base*: good decisions are based on having sufficient objective, accurate and timely information on costs, timescales, benefits and risks. However, projects are too often planned and evaluated on poorly thought-through data and modelling.
- *Stakeholders*: successful projects are driven by the effective interaction of organisations and people who may have widely varying aspirations and requirements. Government tends to be optimistic about its ability to align these different views.
- *Behaviour and incentives*: the National Audit Office refers to the notion of 'strategic misrepresentation' – a desire on the part of individuals and groups to protect and boost their own prospects by securing investment in a project.

- *Challenge and accountability*: decision-makers may be inclined to seek short-term recognition and rewards, and are often not in the same role when a project is under way and problems emerge. At the time of writing, there have been 14 care services ministers since 1997.

All of these factors could be said to have shaped the failures of the market model in adult social care but underpinning them all is policy status. The long-running marginal policy status of adult social care has meant that there were few political constraints on the idea of market-based reforms when it was proposed in the 1980s. Adult social care was not a member of the positive state welfare institutions that joined the general taxation-funded core in the post-war 'golden age'. This has been the underpinning of its fate. Policymakers have consistently failed to move away from a residual funding model towards a more sustainable approach; in this way, the sector has lacked 'path-dependent' mechanisms that tend to automatically increase funding over time (Pierson, 1994).

Unlike universal public subsistence and 'golden age' benefits in kind (notably, the NHS), adult social care has been treated as a marginalised and means-tested model. Chapter 8 noted how the COVID-19 pandemic reinforced rather than challenged this settlement. Indeed, as expenditure policies have tightened, these more 'path-dependent' services have tended to crowd out adult social care. Timmins (1995), for example, notes that in the 1940s, local authority-run provision consisted in the main of what was left over after Nye Bevan had removed many health functions from local authorities for the centralised NHS, and James Griffiths (the social security minister) had made national assistance a national, not a local, responsibility. Today, this marginal status is also seen in the way adult social care is routinely treated as an arm of the NHS rather than a valued service in its own right.

While neoliberalism has found it difficult to reverse some 'golden age' services (especially the NHS), it has been easier to block the evolution of new general taxation-funded welfare state programmes that might increase the relevance, scope, scale and cost of public welfare. This situation has stymied the many proposals and attempts to find an acceptable solution to the funding of long-term care, which, in effect, has never really escaped the Poor Law tradition. This marginal status of the sector has allowed policymakers to aggressively encourage radical, market-based change to the ways in which care is delivered.

This narrow perspective is further reflected in the interpretation of adult social care as 'personal care' rather than as a broader vision of well-being. As noted earlier, the Seebohm Report had a vision of adult social care as a 'universalist' (if not quite a universal) service – 'a door on which anyone could knock' in the words of the report. This position has been repeatedly reduced to one of 'personal care' – support with basic tasks of everyday living, such as washing, dressing and feeding. When the community care legislation was implemented in the 1990s, the idea of a 'social bath' (as opposed to a 'medical bath') was the subject of some derision but it exemplified a crucial delineation between those services that would be provided (free) by the NHS and those provided (subject to a financial assessment) by local authority social services departments (Twigg, 1997).

Despite supporting the idea of free personal care, the Royal Commission on Long Term Care (Sutherland Report, 1999) focused narrowly on the nature of 'personal care', which it defined as all direct care related to: personal toileting, eating and drinking; managing urinary and bowel functions; managing problems associated with mobility and behaviour management; and ensuring personal safety. This understanding excluded costs attributable to such things as cleaning and housework, laundry, shopping services, specialist transport services, and sitting services when the purpose is company or companionship. The commission acknowledged this to be 'on the tight side', yet this conceptualisation has framed the dominant perspective on the nature of adult social care ever since.

This dominant idea of adult social care as a residual means-tested service for those needing assistance with bodily functions is at odds with the newer ideas around 'citizenship' examined in Chapter 8. Citizenship defines those who are – and who are not – members of a common society; it is a manifestly political enterprise (Barbalet, 1988). In his classic text, TH Marshall (1950) described the evolution of citizenship within modernity from the 18th to the 20th century. He argued that it had developed over time, with citizens acquiring civil or market rights in the 18th century, political rights in the 19th century and social rights in the 20th century. For him, the latter were institutionalised in the post-war settlement and the creation of the welfare state. However, unlike civil and political rights, social rights in citizenship require certain distributional activities of the state – they are conditional on the capacity of the fiscal basis of the state to pay for them. However, adult social care has never been a full party to the post-war settlement. Instead, over the last 30 years, the UK has seen the promotion of the narrower notion of the citizen as a customer of public services – 'consumer citizens' with civil or market rights (Daly, 2012).

Making change happen

Any shift from the dominant market model to something approximating the ethical care model set out in Chapter 8 will need support and new ways of thinking. This needs to cover three aspects: practical improvement support; reframing the debate; and challenging established power bases.

Practical improvement support

'Improvement capability' – skills within commissioners and providers, and external support from improvement agencies – is important in helping change to happen. There is a great deal more of this capability in the NHS (especially the hospital sector) than in adult social care, which has never benefited from a fully developed programme to identify and share best practice. Fledgling bodies such as the Care Services Improvement Partnership, the Change Agent Team and the Integrated Care Network became early casualties of the Coalition government's 'quango cull' following the 2010 general election.

Meanwhile, the regulator – the Care Quality Commission – sees its role as primarily one of inspecting and regulating rather than supporting improvement through local relationship building. This is a missed opportunity. A review of the impact of the Care Quality Commission on provider performance (Kings Fund and Manchester University, 2018) emphasised the need for support, not just inspection and regulation. It urged the Care Quality Commission to draw on its intelligence and insight to support providers, foster improvement and prioritise its use of resources. This might involve an inspection workforce with the credibility and skills necessary to foster improvement through close relationships, while maintaining consistency and objectivity. However, this conflation of inspecting and improvement roles is inherently contradictory, and it is likely that improvement support is best delivered by a more trusted 'critical friend'. There seems to have been relatively little attempt to explore these tensions in contemporary institutions, though there is still much to be learned from Henkel's (1991) path-breaking study of the Audit Commission, Social Services Inspectorate and Health Advisory Service. In all three cases, attempts were made to straddle compliance and support to change, sometimes with a degree of success. In each case, it was the perceived independence from government that was vital, allied to credibility within the relevant policy communities.

An interesting recent example of policy support in relation to adult social care is the Care Act 2014 Implementation Support Programme. Given the complexity of the changes introduced by the Care Act, the Department of Health and Social Care and its key partners (the Local Government Association and Association of Directors of Adult Social Services) decided that a comprehensive programme of implementation support should be put in place, both to ensure legislative readiness and to increase the likelihood of smooth implementation. The arrangements involved the establishment of three key organisational innovations – a Programme Board, a Delivery Board and a Programme Management Office – alongside regional infrastructure. The latter – in effect, a time-limited regional improvement support agency – proved to be especially valuable. The regional leads were left free to determine their own ways of working and were well placed to circulate knowledge and secure local authority 'buy-in'. An evaluation of the programme concluded that this regional tier ended up having a significance that far exceeded expectations. Where they worked well, the regional leads were highly regarded, with expressions such as 'the driving force' and 'breathing life' into the implementation process being used (Peckham et al, 2020).

Implicit in all of this is the idea that change needs to happen locally and at the micro level. The role at the national level is to promote and facilitate local change, whereas currently local change movements are often fighting against the grain of national policy. The ideas for an ethical approach to adult social care outlined in Chapter 7 are already being applied in places but tend to exist in isolated pockets rather than being seen as core business. The problem here is not so much a lack of innovation as finding ways for such approaches to take root more deeply in more places. Time, space and resources will be needed to breathe more life into better ways of thinking about service design and delivery; otherwise, the established narrative around access, eligibility and service models will continue to dominate. An important component here will be the need to 'reframe the debate'.

Reframing the debate

Adult social care is uniformly talked about as being 'in crisis' and the dominant narrative has become one of finding the money to meet a growing and unaffordable cost. In 2019, the new Prime Minister, Boris Johnson, joined a long line of politicians (going back to Tony Blair in 1997) who defined the adult social care problem as 'removing the fear of selling your house to pay for care' in older age. This is an extremely narrow frame of reference.

Rather than looking at it in terms of people's lives, social care is spoken of as 'a sector' (or even an 'industry') and a cause of unsustainable pressure on the NHS. The Care Act 2014 – developed on a consensual basis – offered a vision and legislative framework for well-being, with personalised, community-based care and support being the means to those ends. In the event, the focus on funding sidelined the crucial question of what care and support should *do*, as well as of how it needs to work. Too easily, the debate around what a positive vision for the quality of life we would want for ourselves or for our family has been sidelined.

One of the most sustained attempts to capture the narrowness of the current debate and articulate an alternative narrative has been that undertaken by the Social Care Futures movement (Social Care Futures, 2019). Table 5 encapsulates the gaps between the dominant discourse and the alternative vision.

In turn, what this raises is the issue of how the reframing of an issue comes about. Johnson et al (2006) usefully identify four stages in the legitimation process:

- *Stage 1: innovation.* In the first stage, a social innovation is created to address some need, purpose, goal or desire at the local level of actors, such as small groups developing new ways of thinking to accomplish their tasks. Some new objects never acquire legitimacy, whereas others successfully become part of the broader cultural landscape, readily available to others outside of the local context.
- *Stage 2: local validation.* For an innovation to be accepted locally, local actors must construe it as consonant with, and linked to, the existing widely accepted cultural framework of beliefs, values and norms. As a result of being successfully justified (or implicitly accepted), the innovation acquires local validation.
- *Stage 3: diffusion.* Once a new prototype is locally validated, it may be diffused into other new, local situations, and becomes a useful (even necessary) cultural schema for making sense of how things are done. As the new social object spreads, its adoption in new situations often needs less explicit justification than it may have needed in the first local context in which it was adopted.
- *Stage 4: general validation.* Early adopters of an innovation tend to be driven by technical concerns, whereas later adopters can be driven by the legitimacy that comes from emulation. Over time, actors eventually take on the belief that most actors believe that the innovation is acceptable, and once this occurs, the new social object acquires widespread acceptance.

It is hard to say exactly where the reframing of the adult social care discourse has reached in terms of these four stages. Public discourse is still narrow in understanding (Corpus Approaches to Social Science, 2020). An examination of representations of ageing (Centre for Ageing Better, 2020) revealed largely negative understandings, depicted as a 'demographic time bomb', and the positioning of older people as high in warmth but low in competence, in decline and dependent. Although a shift towards more positive representations was appearing to be under way, this was still work in slow progress.

There is certainly much evidence of pockets of innovation and, in some cases, of local validation; however, there remains much still to

Table 5: Dominant and alternative discourses in adult social care

The dominant discourse	The alternative discourse
Vulnerable people looked after by regulated personal care services delivered by care staff: paternalism	People of equal worth leading lives of value that they choose to lead as part of a reciprocal web of community-based support: mutuality
A focus on the challenges faced by 'the sector' in delivering care as a service to people	A focus on people and communities benefiting from, and contributing to, care
Social care is a safety net	Social care is a springboard
People have needs	People have gifts and potential
Social care is in crisis and funding to maintain the status quo is the answer	There are better ideas on how to support people to lead good lives; these require a reformed approach and financial investment
The system needs to be shored up by plugging the current gaps	Sustainable change is needed
National government is the only active agent and needs to fund care	Care and support is co-produced and requires investment
There is growing concern regarding the social and financial cost to society of meeting demand for basic social care	There is growing understanding of the value to society of good care and support
Demand from older and disabled people for social care is a growing and irresolvable pressure on society's resources	By prioritising social care and reforming our approach, we can all reap the dividend of living longer lives
Social care is for older, disabled people and vulnerable adults	Everyone stands to benefit
It is rooted in paternalism regarding those receiving or requiring support, and fairness with respect to funding questions	It is rooted in social justice, equality and rights

Source: Social Care Futures (2019)

do before the final two stages could be said to have been reached. The debate is often expressed as one of securing a 'paradigm shift', an issue discussed in the classic text by Thomas Kuhn (1970) on *The Structure of Scientific Revolutions*. Kuhn sees five key elements to the process of paradigm change: the idea of normal science and received beliefs; the discovery of anomalies and the failure of existing rules; the search and struggle for an alternative paradigm; the process of paradigmatic change; and the establishment of a new paradigm.

As argued earlier, the prime policy dilemma facing adult social care is its capture within the 'path dependency' framework – it has never really been treated as anything much more than a residual means-tested service by policymakers. Although path dependency is a powerful analytical framework, it leans heavily on the claim that events are inevitably repeatable and recurrent, whereas the reality is that history does not repeat itself; rather, it occurs only once in a certain context and at a certain time. In this sense, the model is better at explaining stability than understanding change, yet change is clearly taking place within adult social care (Kay, 2005). An alternative view is that a new paradigm can derive from a supplanted paradigm – a situation where only the more extravagant claims of the old paradigms are contested. The idea of changing *in whole or in part* is important, with the possibility that the new paradigm is offered as part of a suite of options that incorporates the existing paradigm. In effect, this is a suggestion that evolution rather than revolution will be the way in which change is brought about.

This might be especially important in the early phase of paradigmatic war, when the emerging paradigm still contains many uncertainties that can only be answered as progress is achieved. Arguably, this is where the debate on the nature of adult social care is currently situated. The market-based paradigm is deeply entrenched and national politicians show little inclination to think beyond tinkering with this established model. At the same time, there are strong motivations for change at local and grass-roots level, and a willingness to use the experiences arising from this to directly challenge the status quo. The extent to which only the worst problems of marketisation are addressed, rather than a questioning of the model itself, will be a key feature of future debate and direction.

What this debate boils down to is the battle for supremacy between the three key modes of the coordination of social life: markets, hierarchies and networks. This volume has charted the jostling for supremacy between the two best-known approaches – hierarchy and market – as they have been applied to adult social care. Policy has shifted from a largely philanthropic base, to one in which the state offered support along strictly hierarchical and bureaucratic lines expressed through eligibility criteria, and then to a situation in which the market was increasingly seen as a solution. Importantly, these are not seen as mutually exclusive; rather, all have coexisted and what is vital is the balance between them. In turn, this raises the fundamental question of the location of power within and across our current model of adult social care.

Challenging established power bases

Changes to this situation will ultimately be dependent upon changes to the social-structural context within which it operates. In turn, this requires thinking about where power lies in the policymaking process. In his classic analysis of power, Steven Lukes (2005) distinguishes between 'three faces of power': *issue* (power as a relation among people); *agenda* (subtle use of power within a complex system); and *manipulation* (the power to control what people think of as being right). All have been shown to habituate the landscape of adult social care policy in the UK over the past 30 years (Hudson, 2019).

Issue is the 'open face' of power – the ability of one person or group to achieve compliance by openly making decisions that must be observed. In the case of parliamentary legislation, there is at least some basis for this in democratic consent. It is here that the marketisation of adult social care has been built up through key policy landmarks, such as the NHS and Community Care Act 1990 and the Care Act 2014. A shift away from a market model will correspondingly require fresh legislation, as would any serious attempt to shift power towards people who need support, along with promoting alternative modes of sustaining people's independence and well-being.

Agenda is the 'secretive face' of power – the ability to set the agenda and make decisions behind closed doors. This is a situation where it is unclear who is making decisions and on what basis. This has increasingly become the modus operandi of adult social care decision-making, where critical judgements are made without taking into account the needs, views and wishes of those most affected by them. This includes: organisational decisions, such as tightening eligibility criteria for accessing support; professional decisions, where front-line staff exercise discretion in how rules are interpreted and implemented; and business decisions, where judgements on the terms and conditions of care workers, on loading a company with debt in order to extract dividends, and on whether or not to terminate market activity are decided in distant boardrooms. A new approach to adult social care would be based upon an 'open' not a 'secretive' face.

Manipulation is the 'deceptive face' – the power to shape and shift values in such a way that the decisions that create benefit and advantage to the powerful party are accepted without serious questioning. In the case of adult social care, there has been a 30-year period within which to promote the concepts of markets, competition, choice and consumerism as self-evident virtues that require no further justification. Where defects in the model become apparent, these are then interpreted as failures of policy implementation rather than of misconceived policy design. The fact that the most heated policy debates are around funding rather than the model of commissioning and provision bears testimony to the force of manipulative power.

The point has now been reached where there is every reason to challenge all of these normally uncontested assumptions – to challenge all of these faces of power. Commissioning from local suppliers would redirect resources from national and transnational companies to local suppliers and populations. Commissioning small would give preferment to community businesses, not-for-profit organisations and agencies with local roots, local presence and local accountability. Commissioning holistically would challenge the orthodoxy of separate organisations pursuing different and distinct objectives, and place primacy on the importance of 'place' and belonging in people's lives. Commissioning personally would replace the restrictive interpretation of a personal budget with a wider understanding based upon personal outcomes and supported, inclusive communities. Finally, commissioning ethically would offer the opportunity to prioritise non-market values in decision-making to support the social, economic and environmental well-being of an area.

It is important not to simplify the discussion on this balance by taking an entrenched position on the superiority of one over another. Thompson et al (1994) point out that there is not even a single and totally accepted view of how any of these models work. Each will have advantages and downsides:

- Markets will prioritise 'consumer sovereignty' by using the price system to allow consumers to choose how they will deploy their spending power. The application of this approach to adult social care via personal budgets and its earlier variants is one that continues to divide opinion.

- The term 'hierarchy' conjures up ideas of an overweening bureaucracy and impersonal procedural configurations but it also has advantages, such as: reducing arbitrariness in decision-making; treating people according to a set of clear rules; promoting the consistency of decision-making; and enabling greater accountability to be generated. As long as much adult social care is funded by public money, this will remain an important strand.
- A network conjures up the idea of informal high-trust relationships between essentially equal social agents and agencies. Network-based approaches are currently seen as a new and attractive option but how these can be generated, sustained and scaled is still far from clear.

The dilemma for adult social care is that all three of these models are currently in operation in complex, interdependent and sometimes contradictory ways. Reconciling them in ways that help to sustain choice, ensure fairness and generate community connectedness is the task that awaits politicians, policymakers, practitioners, users and communities. Essentially: markets are going where there is money to be made; voluntary endeavour is thriving only where people have the time and inclination to contribute; local authorities are commissioning hand to mouth and on a shoestring; and communities are struggling to find the wherewithal to strengthen bonds. Addressing this complexity will require political determination and excellence in statecraft, neither of which has been much in evidence for over 50 years.

References

ADASS (Association of Directors of Adult Social Services) (2018) *Autumn Budget 2018 – Representation by The Association Of Directors Of Adult Social Services*, London: ADASS. Available at: https://www.adass.org.uk/media/6434/adass-budget-survey-report-2018.pdf

ADASS (2020) *ADASS Coronavirus Survey*, London: ADASS. Available at: https://www.adass.org.uk/media/7973/no-embargo-adass-budget-survey-report.pdf

Age UK (2018) *Behind the Headlines: The Battle to Get Care at Home*, London: Age UK. Available at: http://allcatsrgrey.org.uk/wp/download/social_care/rb_jun18_-the_struggle_to_get_care_at_home.pdf

Age UK (2019) *General Election Manifesto, 2019*, London: Age UK. Available at: https://www.ageuk.org.uk/globalassets/age-uk/documents/campaigns/ge-2019/age-uk-general-election-manifesto-2019.pdf

Allan, T., Thomson, S., Filsak, L. and Ellis, C. (2014) *Evaluation of the Care Certificate Pilot*, London: Skills for Care.

All-Party Parliamentary Group on Social Care (2019) *Elevation, Registration and Standardisation: The Professionalisation of Social Care Workers*, London. Available at: https://img1.wsimg.com/blobby/go/c6219939-c33a-4460-a71e-4df262903498/downloads/SC%20Inquiry%20Final%20%20.pdf

All-Party Parliamentary Group on Social Integration (2020) *Social Connection in the COVID-19 Crisis*, London. Available at: http://www.britishfuture.org/wp-content/uploads/2020/05/Social-Connection-in-the-COVID-19-Crisis.pdf

All-Party Parliamentary Group on Wellbeing Economics (2019) *A Spending Review to Increase Wellbeing*, London. Available at: https://wellbeingeconomics.co.uk/wp-content/uploads/2019/05/Spending-review-to-ncrease-wellbeing-APPG-2019.pdf

Alton, A. (2016) *The Living Wage: Facts and Figures*, Edinburgh: Scottish Parliament. Available at: https://www.parliament.scot/ResearchBriefingsAndFactsheets/S5/SB_16-94_The_Living_Wage_facts_and_figures.pdf

Amnesty International (2020) *As If Expendable: The UK Government's Failure to Protect Older People in Care Homes during the Covid-19 Pandemic*, Available at: https://www.amnesty.org.uk/files/2020-10/Care%20Homes%20Report.pdf?kd5Z8eWzj8Q6ryzHkcaUnxfCtqe5Ddg6=

Association for Public Service Excellence (2018) *Bringing Order to Chaos*, London. Available at: https://www.apse.org.uk/apse/index.cfm/research/apse-direct/2018/marchapril/ad-marchapril/

Association of Directors of Adult Social Services (2018) *Annual Budget Survey 2018*, London. Available at: https://www.adass.org.uk/media/6434/adass-budget-survey-report-2018.pdf

Association of Directors of Adult Social Services (2020) *Adult Social Care: Shaping a Better Future*, London. Available at: https://www.adass.org.uk/media/8036/adult-social-care-shaping-a-better-future-nine-statements-220720.pdf

Association of School and College Leaders (2019) *Navigating the Educational Moral Maze: The Final Report of the Ethical Leadership Commission*, Available at: https://www.nga.org.uk/getattachment/Knowledge-Centre/Good-governance/Ethical-governance/Framework-for-Ethical-Leadership-in-Education/ELC-final-report-jan-19.pdf?lang=en-GB

Audit Commission (1986) *Making a Reality of Community Care*, London: HMSO.

Audit Commission (2004) *Choice in Public Services*, London: HMSO.

Bailey, R. and Brake, M. (1975) *Radical Social Work*, London: Edward Arnold.

Baird, B., Cream, J. and Weaks, L. (2018) *Commissioner Perspectives on Working with the Voluntary, Community and Social Enterprise Sector*, London: King's Fund. Available at: https://www.kingsfund.org.uk/sites/default/files/2018-02/Commissioner_perspectives_on_working_with_the_voluntary_community_and_social_enterprise_sector_1.pdf

Banks, J., Batty, G.D., Coughlin, K., Deepchand, K., Marmot, M., Nazroo, J., Oldfield, Z., Steel, N., Steptoe, A., Wood, M. and Zaninotto, P. (2019) English Longitudinal Study of Ageing: waves 0–8, 1998–2017, data collection, 29th edn, UK Data Service.

Banks, S. (2012) *Ethics and Values in Social Work*, Basingstoke: Palgrave Macmillan.

Barbalet, J.M. (1988) *Citizenship*, Milton Keynes: Open University Press.

Barclay, P. (1982) *Social Workers: Their Role and Tasks*, London: National Institute for Social Work.

Barnes, D., Boland, B., Linhart, K. and Wilson, K. (2017) Personalisation and social care assessment–the Care Act 2014, *BJ Psych Bulletin,* 41(3): 176-80.

Baxter, K., Heavey, E. and Birks, Y. (2019) Choice and control in social care: experiences of older self-funders in England, *Social Policy & Administration*, 54: 460-80.

Baxter, K., Wilberforce, M. and Birks, Y. (2020) What skills do older self-funders in England need to arrange and manage social care? Findings from a scoping review of the Literature, *British Journal of Social Work*, bcaa102, https://doi.org/10.1093/bjsw/bcaa102.

Bedford, S. and Harper, A. (2018) *Sustainable Social Care: What Role for Community Business?*, New Economics Foundation. Available at: https://neweconomics.org/uploads/files/Sustainable-social-care.pdf

Bell, D., Comas-Herrera, A., Henderson, D., Jones, S., Lemmon, E., Moro, M., Murphy, S., O'Reilly, D. and Patrignani, P. (2020) *COVID-19 Mortality and Long Term Care: A UK Comparison*, LTCcovid.org, International Long-Term Care Policy Network, CPEC-LSE, August. Available at: https://ltccovid.org/2020/08/28/covid-19-mortality-and-long-term-care-a-uk-comparison/

Benbow, S. (2008) Failures in the system: our inability to learn from inquiries, *Journal of Adult Protection*, 10(3): 5–13.

Bew, P. (2015) The Committee on Standards in Public Life: twenty years of the Nolan Principles 1995–2015, *Political Quarterly*, 86(3): 411-18.

Bhattacharya, A. (2020) *When and Why Might Choice in Public Services have Intrinsic Value?*, London: Centre for Analysis in Social Exclusion, London School of Economics. Available at: https://sticerd.lse.ac.uk/dps/case/cp/casepaper220.pdf

Birmingham University (2019) *Asset-Based Models: Birmingham University's ICECAP-A Measurement Tool*. Available at: https://www.birmingham.gov.uk/downloads/file/7926/example_of_an_asset_based_approach_-_bartley_green

Birrell, I (2020) *Old Money*, Tortoise. Available at: https://tortoisemedia.com/2020/05/18/coronavirus-care-homes-ian-birrell/

Bolton, J. (2020) *Surviving the Pandemic: New Challenges for Adult Social Care and the Social Care Market*, Institute of Public Care. Available at: https://ipc.brookes.ac.uk/publications/ASC%20Surviving%20the%20Pandemic.pdf

Bottery, S. (2019) *What's Your Problem, Social Care? The Eight Key Areas for Reform*, London: King's Fund. Available at: https://www.kingsfund.org.uk/publications/whats-your-problem-social-care

Bottery, S. and Babalola, G. (2020) *Social Care 360*, London: King's Fund. Available at: https://www.kingsfund.org.uk/publications/social-care-360

Brereton, M. and Temple, M. (1999) The new public service ethos: An ethical environment for governance, *Public Administration,* 77(3): 455–474.

British Academy (2018) *Reforming Business for the 21ˢᵗ Century.* Available at: https://www.legislation.gov.uk/ukpga/2011/20/contents/enacted

British Association of Social Workers (2012) *The Code of Ethics for Social Work.* Available at: https://www.basw.co.uk/about-basw/code-ethics

British Association of Social Workers (2019) *The Anti-poverty Practice Guide for Social Work.* Available at: https://www.basw.co.uk/system/files/resources/Anti%20Poverty%20Guide%20A42.pdf

Broad, R. (2012) *Independent Living: A Cross-Government Strategy About Independent Living for Disabled People,* Centre for Welfare Reform.

Broadhurst, S. and Landau, K. (2017) Learning disability market position statements, are they fit for purpose?, *Tizard Learning Disability Review,* 22(4): 198–205.

Brown, G., Burch, D. and Todd, M. (2019) *Community Business and Anchor Institutions,* Centre for Local Economic Strategies. Available at: https://cles.org.uk/wp-content/uploads/2019/02/Community-business-and-anchor-institutions-Digital.pdf

Brown, L. and Jacobs, L. (2008) *The Private Abuse of the Public Interest,* Chicago, IL: University of Chicago Press.

Buchanan, J. and Tullock, G. (1962) *The Calculus of Consent: Logical Foundations of Constitutional Democracy,* Ann Arbor, MI: University of Michigan Press.

Burns, D., Hyde, P. and Killett, A. (2016) How financial cutbacks affect job quality and the care of the elderly, *Industrial Labour Relations Review,* 69(4): 991–1016.

Burn, E. and Needham, C. (2020) *Implementing the Care Act 2014 – A Synthesis of Project Reports on the Care Act Commissioned by the Policy Research Programme,* University of Birmingham.

Button, D. and Bedford, S. (2019) *Ownership in Social Care: Why It Matters and What Can Be Done,* London: New Economics Foundation. Available at: https://neweconomics.org/uploads/files/Ownership-in-social-care-report.pdf

Callaghan, J. (2014) Professions and professionalization, in T. Teo (ed) *Encyclopedia of Critical Psychology,* New York, NY: Springer.

Campbell, J. and Oliver, M. (1996) *Disability Politics: Understanding Our Past, Changing Our Future,* London: Routledge.

Care Quality Commission (2014) *A Fresh Start for the Regulation and Inspection of Adult Social Care,* London. Available at: https://www.cqc.org.uk/sites/default/files/documents/20131013_cqc_afreshstart_2013_final.pdf

Care Quality Commission (2017a) *The State of the Adult Social Care Services 2014–17*. Available at: https://www.cqc.org.uk/sites/default/files/20170703_ASC_end_of_programme_FINAL2.pdf

Care Quality Commission (2017b) *State of Care, 2016/17*, London. Available at: https://www.cqc.org.uk/sites/default/files/20171123_stateofcare1617_report.pdf

Care Quality Commission (2019) *The State of Health Care and Adult Social Care in England 2018/19*. Available at: https://www.cqc.org.uk/sites/default/files/20191015b_stateofcare1819_fullreport.pdf

Care Quality Commission (2020) *Out of Sight – Who Cares? A Review of Restraint, Seclusion and Segregation for Autistic People, and People with a Learning Disability and/or Mental Health Condition*. Available at: https://www.cqc.org.uk/sites/default/files/20201218_rssreview_report.pdf

Carers UK (2019a) *State of Caring Survey*. Available at: http://www.carersuk.org/images/News__campaigns/CUK_State_of_Caring_2019_Report.pdf

Carers UK (2019b) *Will I Care?*. Available at: https://www.carersuk.org/images/News__campaigns/CarersRightsDay_Nov19_FINAL.pdf

Carey, G., Malbon, E., Green, C., Reeders, D. and Marjolin, A. (2020) Quasi-market shaping, stewarding and steering in personalization: the need for practice-orientated empirical evidence, *Policy Design and Practice*, 3(1): 30-44.

Carey, M. (2015) The fragmentation of social work and social care: some ramifications and a critique, *The British Journal of Social Work*, 45(8): 2406–22.

Carr, S. (2013) *Improving Personal Budgets for Older People: A Research Overview*, Social Care Institute for Excellence. Available at: https://www.scie.org.uk/publications/reports/report63.asp

Cavendish Review (2013) *An Independent Review into Healthcare Assistants and Support Workers in the NHS and Social Care Settings*, London. Available at: https://assets.publishing.service.gov.uk/government/uploads/system/uploads/attachment_data/file/236212/Cavendish_Review.pdf

Centre for Ageing Better (2020) *An Old Age Problem? How society shapes and reinforces negative attitudes to ageing*. Available at; https://www.ageing-better.org.uk/publications/old-age-problem-how-society-shapes-and-reinforces-negative-attitudes-ageing

Centre for Local Economic Strategies (2018) *Restoring Public Values in Public Services*, Manchester. Available at: https://cles.org.uk/publications/restoring-public-values-in-public-services/

Centre for Local Economic Studies (2020) *Understanding and Diversifying Care Markets*.

Centre for Local Economic Studies (2020) *A Progressive Approach to Adult Social Care*. Available at: https://cles.org.uk/publications/a-progressive-approach-to-adult-social-care/

Centre for Progressive Policy (2020) *A Gear Change for Growth*. Available at: https://www.progressive-policy.net/downloads/files/CPP_A-gear-change-for-growth.pdf

Centre for Research on Socio-Cultural Change (2016) *Public Interest Report: Where Does the Money Go? Financialised Chains and the Crisis in Residential Care*. Available at: https://hummedia.manchester.ac.uk/institutes/cresc/research/WDTMG%20FINAL%20-01-3-2016.pdf

Centre for Social Justice (2020) *Coronavirus and Voluntary Sector Resilience. Available at: https://www.centreforsocialjustice.org.uk/core/wp-content/uploads/2020/03/Covid-19_Publication_v3.pdf*

Charity Commission for England and Wales (2020) *Charity Commission Annual Report 2019-20*. Available at: https://assets.publishing.service.gov.uk/government/uploads/system/uploads/attachment_data/file/901690/Charity_Commission_Annual_Report_and_Accounts_2019_to_2020.pdf

CHPI (Centre for Health and the Public Interest) (2013) *The Future of the NHS? Lessons from the Market in Social Care in England*. Available at: https://chpi.org.uk/wp-content/uploads/2013/10/CHPI-Lessons-from-the-social-care-market-October-2013.pdf

CHPI (2019) *Plugging the Leaks in the UK Care Home Industry*. Available at: https://chpi.org.uk/wp-content/uploads/2019/11/CHPI-PluggingTheLeaks-Nov19-FINAL.pdf

Clarke, J. (2006) Consumers, clients or citizens? Politics, policy and practice in the reform of social care, *European Societies*, 8(3): 423–42.

Comas-Herrera, A., Salcher-Konrad, M., Baumbusch, J., Farina, N., Goodman, C., Lorenz-Dant, K. and Low, L.-F. (2020), *Rapid Review of the Evidence on Impacts of Visiting Policies in Care Homes During the Covid-19 Pandemic*, LTCcovid.org. Available at: https://ltccovid.org/2020/11/01/pre-print-rapid-review-of-the-evidence-on-impacts-of-visiting-policies-in-care-homes-during-the-covid-19-pandemic/

Commission on Evidence-Based Policymaking (2017) *Final Report*. Available at: https://www.cep.gov/report/cep-final-report.pdf

Committee on Standards in Public Life (2014) *Ethical Standards for Providers of Public Services*. Available at: https://assets.publishing.service.gov.uk/government/uploads/system/uploads/attachment_data/file/336942/CSPL_EthicalStandards_web.pdf

Committee on Standards in Public Life (2018) *The Continuing Importance of Ethical Standards for Public Services Providers*. Available at: https://assets.publishing.service.gov.uk/government/uploads/system/uploads/attachment_data/file/705884/20180510_PSP2_Final_PDF.pdf

Commons Digital, Culture, Media and Sports Committee (2020) *The COVID-19 Crisis and Charities*. Available at: https://committees.parliament.uk/publications/938/documents/7200/default/

Commons Health and Social Care Committee (2020) *Social Care: Funding and Workforce*. Available at: https://publications.parliament.uk/pa/cm5801/cmselect/cmhealth/206/20602.htm

Commons Public Accounts Committee (2020a) *Whole of Government Response to Covid-19*. Available at: https://publications.parliament.uk/pa/cm5801/cmselect/cmpubacc/404/40402.htm

Commons Public Accounts Committee (2020b), *Readying the NHS and Social Care for the Covid-19 Peak*. Available at: https://committees.parliament.uk/work/345/readying-the-nhs-and-social-care-for-the-covid19-peak/publications/

Commons Public Administration and Constitutional Affairs Committee (2018) After Carillion: Public sector outsourcing and contracting, HC 748. Available at: https://publications.parliament.uk/pa/cm201719/cmselect/cmpubadm/748/748.pdf

Commons Science and Technology Committee (2016) *Forensic Science Strategy Inquiry*. Available at: https://publications.parliament.uk/pa/cm201617/cmselect/cmsctech/501/501.pdf

Commons Women and Equalities Committee (2020) *Unequal Impact: Coronavirus, Disability and Access to Services: Interim Report on Temporary Provisions in the Coronavirus Act*. Available at: https://committees.parliament.uk/publications/2710/documents/27010/default/

Community Care (Direct Payments) Act (1996) London: The Stationery Office. Available at: https://www.legislation.gov.uk/ukpga/1996/30/contents

Community Catalysts (2018) Home page. Available at: www.communitycatalysts.co.uk/

Competition and Markets Authority (2017) *Care Homes Market Study: Final Report*. Available at: https://assets.publishing.service.gov.uk/media/5a1fdf30e5274a750b82533a/care-homes-market-study-final-report.pdf

Competition and Markets Authority (2018) *Care Homes: Consumer Law Advice for Providers*. Available at: https://assets.publishing.service.gov.uk/government/uploads/system/uploads/attachment_data/file/759257/Care_homes_full_guidance_for_providers.pdf

Consilium and Skills for Care (2016) *Study into the Impact of a Values Based Approach to Recruitment and Retention*. Available at: https://www.skillsforcare.org.uk/Documents/NMDS-SC-and-intelligence/Research-evidence/Values-based-recruitment-Final-evaluation-report.pdf

Cooper, C., Marston, L., Barber, J., Livingston, D., Rapaport, P., Higgs, D. and Livingston, G. (2018) Do care homes deliver person-centred care? A cross-sectional survey of staff-reported abusive and positive behaviours towards residents from the MARQUE (Managing Agitation and Raising Quality of Life) English national care home survey, *Plos One*, March. Available at: https://pubmed.ncbi.nlm.nih.gov/29561867/

Cooperative Party (2018) *Democratic Public Ownership for the 21st Century*. Available at: https://party.coop/policy/ownership-matters/summary/

Corlett, A. and Gardiner, L. (2018) *Home Affairs: Options for Reforming Property Taxation*, Resolution Foundation. Available at: https://www.resolutionfoundation.org/app/uploads/2018/03/Council-tax-IC.pdf

Coronavirus Act (2020) London: The Stationery Office. Available at: https://www.legislation.gov.uk/ukpga/2020/7/contents/enacted

Corpus Approaches to Social Science (2020) *Social Care in UK Public Discourse*, University of Lancaster. Available at: http://cass.lancs.ac.uk/wp-content/uploads/2020/04/CASS-BRIEFING-14-Social-Care.pdf

Corrigan, P. and Leonard, P. (1978) *Social Work under Capitalism*, London: Macmillan.

Corry, D. (2020) *Where Are England's Charities?*, London: New Philanthropy Capital. Available at: https://www.thinknpc.org/resource-hub/where-are-englands-charities/

CSI Market Intelligence (2020) *Say Hello, Wave Goodbye: Openings and Closures of Care Homes for Older People, 2019*. Available at: https://csi-marketintelligence.co.uk/#sayhello

Cumbers, A. and Hanna, T. (2019) *Constructing the Democratic Public Enterprise*, Democracy Collaborative, University of Glasgow. Available at: https://democracycollaborative.org/sites/default/files/2020-02/Constructing%20the%20Democratic%20Public%20Enterprise.pdf

Curry, N., Schlepper, L. and Hemmings, N. (2019) *What Can England Learn from the Long-Term Care System in Germany?*, Nuffield Trust. Available at: https://www.nuffieldtrust.org.uk/files/2019-12/ltci-germany-br1924-6-web.pdf

Daly, G. (2012) Citizenship, choice and care: an examination of the promotion of choice in the provision of adult social care, *Research, Policy and Planning*, 29(3): 179–89.

Davey, V., Fernández, J.L., Knapp, M., Vick, N., Jolly, D., Swift, P., Tobin, R., Kendall, J., Ferrie, J., Pearson, C., Mercer, G. and Preistley, M. (2007) *Direct Payments: A National Survey of Direct Payments Policy and Practice*, London: PSSRU and London School of Economics. Available at: https://www.pssru.ac.uk/pub/dprla.pdf

Davies, K., Dalgarno, E., Davies, S., Roberts, A., Hughes, J., Chester, H., Jasper, R., Wilson, D. and Challis, D. (2020) *The challenges of commissioning home care for older people in England: commissioners' perspective*, University of Nottingham. https://nottingham-repository.worktribe.com/output/3839737/the-challenges-of-commissioning-home-care-for-older-people-in-england-commissioners-perspectives

Deakin, N. (1994) *The Politics of Welfare: Continuity and Change*, London: Harvester Wheatsheaf.

Deloitte-NZ (2018) *Beyond GDP Measuring New Zealand's Wellbeing Progress*. Available at: https://www2.deloitte.com/content/dam/Deloitte/nz/Documents/public-sector/Deloitte-NZ-SotS-2018-Article-2.pdf

Department of Health (1989) *Caring for People: Community Care in the Next Decade and Beyond*, London: HMSO.

Department of Health (2003) *Fair Access to Care Services: Guidance on Eligibility Criteria for Adult Social Care*, London: HMSO.

Department of Health (2007) *Putting People First: A Shared Vision and Commitment to the Transformation of Adult Social Care*, London: HMSO.

Department of Health (2012) *Market Oversight in Adult Social Care*, London: HMSO. Available at: https://assets.publishing.service.gov.uk/government/uploads/system/uploads/attachment_data/file/144207/market-oversight-consultation-document.pdf

Department of Health (2013) *Strengthening Corporate Accountability in Health and Social Care*, London: HMSO. Available at: https://assets.publishing.service.gov.uk/government/uploads/system/uploads/attachment_data/file/210734/Corporate_accountability.pdf

Department of Health (2014) *Strengthening Corporate Accountability in Health and Social Care: Consultation on the Fit and Proper Person Regulations*, London: HMSO. Available at:https://assets.publishing.service.gov.uk/government/uploads/system/uploads/attachment_data/file/298328/Corporate_accountability_consultation_response..pdf

Department of Health (2016) *Care and Continuity: Contingency Planning for Provider Failure*, London: HMSO. Available at: https://www.basw.co.uk/system/files/resources/basw_105421-4_0.pdf

Department of Health and Social Care (2018a) *Care and Support: Statutory Guidance*, London: HSMO. Available at: https://www.gov.uk/government/publications/care-act-statutory-guidance/care-and-support-statutory-guidance

Department of Health and Social Care (2018b) *Government Response to the CMA Care Homes Market Study, Final Report*, London: HMSO. Available at: https://assets.publishing.service.gov.uk/government/uploads/system/uploads/attachment_data/file/685315/cma-care-homes-market-study-final-report-government-response.pdf

Department of Health and Social Care (2020a) *Our Action Plan for Adult Social Care*, London: HMSO. Available at: https://www.gov.uk/government/publications/coronavirus-covid-19-adult-social-care-action-plan/covid-19-our-action-plan-for-adult-social-care

Department of Health and Social Care (2020b) *Responding to COVID-19: The Ethical Framework for Adult Social Care*, London: HMSO. Available at: https://www.gov.uk/government/publications/covid-19-ethical-framework-for-adult-social-care/responding-to-covid-19-the-ethical-framework-for-adult-social-care

Department of Health and Social Care (2020c) *Care Act Easements: Guidance for Local Authorities*, London: HMSO. Available at: https://www.gov.uk/government/publications/coronavirus-covid-19-changes-to-the-care-act-2014/care-act-easements-guidance-for-local-authorities

Department of Health and Social Care (2020d) *Social Care Sector Covid-19 Support Taskforce: final report, advice and recommendations*, London: HMSO. Available at: *https://www.gov.uk/government/publications/social-care-sector-covid-19-support-taskforce-report-on-first-phase-of-covid-19-pandemic/social-care-sector-covid-19-support-taskforce-final-report-advice-and-recommendations*

Department of Health and Social Care (2020e) *Coronavirus (COVID-19) Action Plan*, London: HMSO. Available at: *https://www.gov.uk/government/publications/coronavirus-covid-19-adult-social-care-action-plan*

Department of Health and Social Care (2020f) *Our Plan to Rebuild: The UK Government's COVID-19 Recovery Strategy*, London: HMSO. Available at: *https://www.gov.uk/government/publications/our-plan-to-rebuild-the-uk-governments-covid-19-recovery-strategy/our-plan-to-rebuild-the-uk-governments-covid-19-recovery-strategy*

Department of Health and Social Care (2020g) *COVID-19: Care Home Support Package,* London: HMSO. Available at: *https://www.gov. uk/government/publications/coronavirus-covid-19-support-for-care-homes/ coronavirus-covid-19-care-home-support-package*

Dilnot Report (2011) *Fairer Funding for All – The Commission's Recommendations to Government,* Commission on Funding of Care and Support. Available at: https://webarchive.nationalarchives.gov. uk/20120713201059/http://www.dilnotcommission.dh.gov.uk/ files/2011/07/Fairer-Care-Funding-Report.pdf

Directory of Social Change (2020) *Over Half of Charities Could Disappear within Six Months.* Available at: https://www.dsc.org.uk/content/ over-half-of-charities-could-disappear-within-6-months/

Dockley, A. and Loader, I. (2016) *The Penal Landscape: The Howard League Guide to Criminal Justice in England and Wales,* London: Howard League for Penal Reform. Available at: https://howardleague.org/ publications/the-penal-landscape-the-howard-league-guide-to-criminal-justice-in-england-and-wales/

Edwards, N. and Kumpunen, S. (2019) *Primary Care Networks: A Pre-Mortem to Identify Potential Risks,* Nuffield Trust. Available at: https://www.nuffieldtrust.org.uk/files/2019-11/ primary-care-networks-final-v3.pdf

Erskine, J., Castelli, M., Hunter, D. and Hungin, P. (2018) The persistent problem of integrated care in English NHS hospitals, *Journal of Health Organisation and Management,* 32(4): 532–44.

Eurofound (2017) *Care Homes for Older Europeans: Public, For-Profit and Non-profit Providers,* Brussels: Eurofound. Available at: https:// www.eurofound.europa.eu/sites/default/files/ef_publication/field_ ef_document/ef1723en.pdf

European Commission (2017) *Commission Recommendation Establishing the European Pillar of Social Rights,* Brussels. Available at: https:// ec.europa.eu/info/publications/commission-recommendation-establishing-european-pillar-social-rights_en

Evans, J. (2003) *The Independent Living Movement in the UK,* Sweden: Independent Living Institute. Available at: https://www. independentliving.org/docs6/evans2003.html

Fair Work Convention (2019) *Fair Work in Scotland's Social Care Sector,* Glasgow: Fair Work Convention. Available at: https://www. fairworkconvention.scot/our-report-on-fair-work-in-social-care/

Fowler, N. (1984) Speech at Association of Directors of Social Services Conference, Buxton.

Fox, A. (2018) *A New Health and Care System: Escaping the Invisible Asylum,* Bristol: Policy Press.

Future Care Capital (2019) *Data That Cares*, London: Future Care Capital. Available at: https://futurecarecapital.org.uk/research/data-that-cares/

Gamble, A. (1988) *The Free Economy and the Strong State*, London: Palgrave.

Gaskell, J., Stoker, G., Jennings, W. and Devine, D. (2020) Covid-19 and the blunders of our governments: Long-run system failings aggravated by political choices, *Political Quarterly*, 91(3): 523-33. Available at: https://onlinelibrary.wiley.com/doi/full/10.1111/1467-923X.12894

Glasby, J., Zhang, Y., Bennett, R. and Hall, P. (2020) A lost decade? A renewed case for adult social care reform in England, *Journal of Social Policy*, August. Available at: https://www.cambridge.org/core/journals/journal-of-social-policy/article/lost-decade-a-renewed-case-for-adult-social-care-reform-in-england/6309C490CD09B4009F3369E2E5AEB1D9

Glennerster, H. (1981) From containment to conflict? Social planning in the seventies, *Journal of Social Policy*, 10(1): 31–51.

Government Commercial Function (2019) *The Outsourcing Playbook: Central Government Guidance on Outsourcing Decisions and Contracting*, London: HMSO. Available at: https://assets.publishing.service.gov.uk/government/uploads/system/uploads/attachment_data/file/891144/Outsourcing_Playbook_JUNE_2020_WEB.pdf

Gray, A. M. and Birrell, D. (2013) *Transforming Adult Social Care: Contemporary Policy and Practice*, Bristol: Policy Press.

Gray, M. and Barford, A. (2018) The depths of the cuts: the uneven geography of local government austerity, *Cambridge Journal of Regions Economy and Society*, 11: 541–563.

Green, D. (2019) *Fixing the Care Crisis*, Centre for Policy Studies. Available at: https://www.cps.org.uk/files/reports/original/190426143506-DamianGreenSocialCareFinal.pdf

Griffiths, R. (1988) *Community Care: Agenda for Action* (Griffiths Report), London: HMSO.

Hadley, R. and Hatch, R. (1981) *Social Welfare and the Failure of the State: Centralised Social Services and Participatory Alternatives*, George Allen and Unwin.

Hall, P. (1976) *Reforming the Welfare: The Politics of Change in the Personal Social Services*, London: Heinemann

Hallett, C. (1982) *The Personal Social Services in Local Government*, London: Allen & Unwin.

Hambleton, R. (2014) *Leading the Inclusive City: Place-Based Innovation for a Bounded Planet*, Bristol: Policy Press.

Hardy, B. and Wistow, G. (2000) Changes in the private sector, in B. Hudson (ed) *The Changing Role of Social Care*, London: Jessica Kingsley.

Hare, R.M. (1952) *The Language of Morals*, Oxford: Clarendon Press.

Harris, T., Hodge, L. and Phillips, D. (2019) *English Local Government Funding: Trends and Challenges in 2019 and Beyond*, London: Institute for Fiscal Studies. Available at: https://www.ifs.org.uk/uploads/ English-local-government-funding-trends-and-challenges-in-2019- and-beyond-IFS-Report-166.pdf

Hayes, L., Tarrant, A. and Walters, H. (2020) *Care and Support Workers' Perceptions of Health and Safety Issues in Social Care during the COVID- 19 Pandemic: Initial Findings*, University of Kent. Available at: https:// media.www.kent.ac.uk/se/11148/CareworkersHealthandSafetyrepo rt15042.pdf

Health Foundation (2020) *Briefing: Adult Social Care and COVID- 19: Assessing the Impact on Social Care Users and Staff in England so Far*, London: The Health Foundation. Available at: https://reader. health.org.uk/adult-social-care-and-covid-19-assessing-the-impact- on-social-care-users-and-staff-in-england-so-far

Health Foundation and King's Fund (2018) *Approaches to Social Care Funding*, Available at: https://www.kingsfund.org.uk/sites/default/ files/2018-03/Approaches-to-social-care-funding.pdf

Health Services and Public Health Act (1968) London: The Stationery Office. Available at: https://www.legislation.gov.uk/ukpga/1968/46

HealthWatch/British Red Cross (2020) *590 People's Stories of Leaving Hospital during Covid-19*. Available at: https://www.healthwatch. co.uk/sites/healthwatch.co.uk/files/20201026%20Peoples%20 experiences%20of%20leaving%20hospital%20during%20COVID- 19_0.pdf

Held, V. (2006) *The Ethics of Care: Personal, Political and Global*, Oxford: Oxford University Press.

Henkel, M. (1991) *Government, Evaluation and Change*, London: Jessica Kingsley.

Henricson, C. (2016) *Morality and Public Policy*, Bristol: Policy Press.

Henwood, M. and Hudson, B. (2008) *Lost to the System: The Impact of Fair Access to Care*, London: Commission for Social Care Inspection. Available at: http://www.melaniehenwood.com/perch/resources/ cscifacslosttothesystem.pdf

Henwood, M., Mckay, S., Needham, C. and Glasby, J. (2018) *From Bystanders to Core Participants: A Literature and Data Review of Self-Funders in Social Care Markets*, University of Birmingham, Health Services Management Centre. Available at: https://www.birmingham.ac.uk/Documents/college-social-sciences/social-policy/HSMC/publications/2018/UoB-PRP-Self-funders-review-of-data-and-literature-FINAL.pdf

HFT (2020) *Sector Pulse Check: The Impact of the Changes to the Social Care Sector in 2019*, Bristol: HFT. Available at: https://www.hft.org.uk/wp-content/uploads/2020/02/Hft-Sector-Pulse-Check-2019.pdf.

HM Government (2013) *Choice Charter,* Available at: https://assets.publishing.service.gov.uk/government/uploads/system/uploads/attachment_data/file/199781/Choice_Charter.pdf

HM Government (2018) *Civil Society Strategy: Building a Future That Works for Everyone.* Available at: https://assets.publishing.service.gov.uk/government/uploads/system/uploads/attachment_data/file/732765/Civil_Society_Strategy_-_building_a_future_that_works_for_everyone.pdf

HM Inspectorate of Probation (2017) *Annual Report, 2017,* Available at: https://www.justiceinspectorates.gov.uk/hmiprobation/wp-content/uploads/sites/5/2017/12/HMI-Probation-Annual-Report-2017-2.pdf

Hollis, F. (1948) *Social Casework in Practice*, New York, NY: Family Service Association of America.

Home Office (2020) *The UK's Points-Based Immigration System: Policy Statement.* Available at: https://www.gov.uk/government/publications/the-uks-points-based-immigration-system-policy-statement/the-uks-points-based-immigration-system-policy-statement

Hood, C. (1991) A public management for all seasons?, *Public Administration*, 69: 3–19.

Hood, C. (1995) Contemporary public management: a new global paradigm?, *Public Policy and Administration*, 10(2): 104–117.

House of Commons Business, Energy and Industrial Strategy Committee and Work and Pensions Committee (2018) *Carillion.* Available at: https://publications.parliament.uk/pa/cm201719/cmselect/cmworpen/769/76902.htm

House of Commons Committee of Public Accounts (2016) *The Sale of Former Northern Rock Assets.* Available at: https://publications.parliament.uk/pa/cm201617/cmselect/cmpubacc/632/632.pdf

House of Commons Committee of Public Accounts (2017) *Personal Budgets in Social Care, Second Report of Session 2016–17*. Available at: https://publications.parliament.uk/pa/cm201617/cmselect/cmpubacc/74/74.pdf

House of Commons Committee of Public Accounts (2019) *Local Government Spending*. Available at: https://publications.parliament.uk/pa/cm201617/cmselect/cmpubacc/74/74.pdf

House of Commons Communities and Local Government Committee (2017) *Adult Social Care*. Available at: https://publications.parliament.uk/pa/cm201617/cmselect/cmcomloc/1103/110303.htm

House of Commons Health and Social Care Committee (2018) *Integrated Care Organisations, Partnerships and Systems, HC 650*. Available at: https://publications.parliament.uk/pa/cm201719/cmselect/cmhealth/650/65002.htm

House of Commons Health Committee (2014) *2013 Accountability Hearing with the Care Quality Commission*. Available at: https://publications.parliament.uk/pa/cm201012/cmselect/cmhealth/1430/1430.pdf

House of Commons Library (2019a) *Four Seasons Health Care Group – Financial Difficulties and Safeguards for Clients, Briefing Paper Number 8004*. Available at: https://commonslibrary.parliament.uk/research-briefings/cbp-8004/

House of Commons Library (2019b) *Adult Social Care: The Government's Ongoing Policy Review and Anticipated Green Paper (England)*. Available at: https://commonslibrary.parliament.uk/research-briefings/cbp-8002/

House of Commons Library (2020a) *Reviewing and Reforming Local Government Finance*. Available at: https://commonslibrary.parliament.uk/research-briefings/cbp-7538/

House of Commons Library (2020b) *Adult Social Care Funding*. Available at: https://commonslibrary.parliament.uk/research-briefings/cbp-7903/

House of Commons Library (2020c) *Coronavirus Bill: Health and Social Care Measures*. Available at: https://commonslibrary.parliament.uk/research-briefings/cbp-8861/

House of Commons Public Accounts Committee (2014) *Adult Social Care in England*, London. Available at: https://publications.parliament.uk/pa/cm201415/cmselect/cmpubacc/518/51802.htm.

House of Commons Public Accounts Committee (2018) *Interface between Health and Adult Social Care*. Available at: https://publications.parliament.uk/pa/cm201719/cmselect/cmpubacc/1376/1376.pdf

House of Commons Social Security Committee (1991) *The Financing of Private Residential and Nursing Home Fees*, London: HMSO.

Huberts, L. (2018) Integrity: what it is and why it is important, *Public Integrity*, 20: 18–32.

Hudson, B. (2011a) Big Society: a concept in pursuit of a definition, *Journal of Integrated Care*, 19(5): 17–24.

Hudson, B. (2011b) Ten years of jointly commissioning health and social care in England, *International Journal of Integrated Care*, 11(special 10th anniversary edn). Available at: https://www.ncbi.nlm.nih.gov/pmc/articles/PMC3111886/

Hudson, B. (2014) Dealing with market failure: a new dilemma in UK health and social care policy?, *Critical Social Policy*, 35(2): 281–92.

Hudson, B. (2019) Commissioning for change: a new model for commissioning adult social care in England, *Critical Social Policy*, 39(3): 413–33.

Hudson, B. and Henwood, M. (2002) The NHS and social care: the final countdown?, *Policy and Politics*, 30(2):153–66.

Hudson, B., Hunter, D. and Peckham, S. (2019) Policy failure and the policy–implementation gap: can policy support programs help?, *Policy Design and Practice*, 2(1): 1–14.

Humphreys, R. (2001) *Poor Relief and Charity 1869–1945*, London: Palgrave Macmillan.

Hunter, D., Hudson, B., Peckham, S. and Redgate, S. (2020) Do policy implementation support programmes work? The case of the Care Act 2014, *Journal of Long-Term Care,* pp196–207. Available at: *https://journal.ilpnetwork.org/articles/10.31389/jltc.42/*

Idriss, O., Allen, L. and Alderwick, H. (2020) *Social Care for Adults Aged 18–64*, London: Health Foundation. Available at: https://www.health.org.uk/publications/reports/social-care-for-adults-aged-18-64

IFC Consulting (2018) *The Economic Value of the Adult Social Care Sector, UK*. Available at: https://www.skillsforcare.org.uk/Documents/About/sfcd/Economic-value-of-the-adult-social-care-sector-UK.pdf

IFG Consulting (2018) *Government Procurement: The Scale and Nature of Contracting in the UK*, London: Institute for Government. Available at: https://www.instituteforgovernment.org.uk/contact-us

Incisive Health (2019) *Care Deserts: The Impact of a Dysfunctional Market in Adult Social Care Provision*. Available at: https://www.ageuk.org.uk/globalassets/age-uk/documents/reports-and-publications/reports-and-briefings/care—support/care-deserts—-age-uk-report.pdf

Independent Age (2019) *Reviewing the Case: The Right to Appeal in Adult Social Care*. Available at: https://independent-age-assets. s3.eu-west-1.amazonaws.com/s3fs-public/2019-10/IA-PI-092-SocialCareAppeals_WEB_0.pdf

Institute for Fiscal Studies (2020) *COVID-19 and English council funding: hit to budgets in 2020–21*. Available at: https://www.ifs. org.uk/uploads/R-174-COVID-19%20and%20English-council-funding-how-are-budgets-being-hit-in-2020%E2%80%9321.pdf

Institute for Government (2019) *Performance Tracker 2019*. Available at: https://www.instituteforgovernment.org.uk/sites/default/files/ publications/performance-tracker-2019_0.pdf

Institute for Local Governance (2018) *How to Work Effectively with the Third Sector*, University of Durham. Available at: https://www. stchads.ac.uk/wp-content/uploads/2018/02/ILG-How-to-work-effectively-with-the-third-sector-discussion-paper-March-2019-.pdf

Institute of Public Care (2014) *The Stability of the Care Market and Market Oversight in England*. Available at: https://www.cqc.org.uk/ sites/default/files/201402-market-stability-report.pdf.

Institute of Public Care (2016) *What Are the Opportunities and Threats for Further Savings in Adult Social Care?* Available at: https://www.scie-socialcareonline.org.uk/what-are-the-opportunities-and-threats-for-further-savings-in-adult-social-care/r/a11G0000009T9d2IAC.

International Long-Term Care Policy Network (2020) *Long-Term Care Responses to COVID-19*. Available at: https://ltccovid.org/ country-reports-on-covid-19-and-long-term-care/

IPPR (Institute for Public Policy Research) (2018a) *Prosperity and Justice: A Plan for the New Economy – The Final Report of the IPPR Commission on Economic Justice*. Available at: https://www.ippr.org/ files/2018-08/1535639099_prosperity-and-justice-ippr-2018.pdf

IPPR (2018b) *Fair Care: A Workforce Strategy for Social Care*, London. Available at: https://www.ippr.org/files/2018-11/fair-care-a-workforce-strategy-november18.pdf

Irwin Mitchell (2020) *Elderly Care Crisis: A Tipping Point*. Available at: https://www.irwinmitchell.com/elderly-care-crisis

Jackson, R. (2018) *Reforming Social Care: Time for Radical Change*, Centre for Welfare Reform. Available at: https://www.centreforwelfarereform. org/uploads/attachment/607/reforming-social-care.pdf

Johnson, C., Dowd, T. and Ridgeway, C. (2006) Legitimacy as a social process, *American Sociological Review*, 32: 53–78.

Johnson, P. (2014) Sociology and the critique of neoliberalism: reflections on Peter Wagner and Axel Honneth, *European Journal of Social Theory*, 17(4): 516–33.

Jones, K. (1972) *A History of the Mental Health Services*, London: Routledge & Kegan Paul.

Jones, K., Forder, J., Welch, E., Caiels, J. and Fox, D. (2017) *Personal Health Budgets: Process and Context Following the National Pilot Programme*, PSSRU and University of Kent. Available at: https://www.pssru.ac.uk/pub/5433.pdf

Jones, R. (2018) *In Whose Interest? The Privatisation of Child Protection and Social Work*, Bristol: Policy Press.

Jones, R. (2020) *A History of the Personal Social Services in England, London:* Palgrave Macmillan.

Just Group (2019) *Care Reform, What Reform?*. Available at: https://www.justgroupplc.co.uk/~/media/Files/J/JRMS-IR/news-doc/2019/2019%20Care%20Report%20-%20what%20reform.pdf

Kay, A. (2005) A critique of the use of path dependency in policy studies, *Public Administration*, 83(3): 553–71.

King's Fund (2018) *Approaches to Social Care Funding*. Available at: https://www.kingsfund.org.uk/publications/approaches-social-care-funding

King's Fund and Manchester University (2018) *Impact of the Care Quality Commission on Provider Performance*. Available at: https://www.kingsfund.org.uk/sites/default/files/2018-09/cqc-provider-performance-report-september2018.pdf

King's Fund, Nuffield Trust and Health Foundation (2019) *Closing the Gap: Key Areas for Action on the Health and Care Workforce*. Available at: https://www.kingsfund.org.uk/sites/default/files/2019-06/closing-the-gap-full-report-2019.pdf

Klinenberg, E. (2018) *Palaces for the People: How to Build a More Equal and United Society*, London: Penguin.

Knight, A., Lowe, T., Brossard, M. and Wilson, J. (2017) *A Whole New World: Funding and Commissioning in Complexity*, Newcastle University Business School. Available at: http://wordpress.collaboratei.com/wp-content/uploads/A-Whole-New-World-Funding-Commissioning-in-Complexity.pdf

Knight Frank (2019) *UK Residential Market Update, June 2019*. Available at: https://content.knightfrank.com/research/100/documents/en/uk-residential-market-update-june-2019-6453.pdf

Knight Frank (2020) *Healthcare Capital Markets 2020*. Available at: https://content.knightfrank.com/research/105/documents/en/healthcare-capital-markets-2020-7029.pdf

Kuhn, T. (1970) *The Structure of Scientific Revolutions*, Chicago, IL: University of Chicago.

Labour Party (2019) *Towards the National Care Service: Labour's Vision*. Available at: https://labour.org.uk/wp-content/uploads/2019/09/12703_19-Towards-the-National-Care-Service.pdf

Laing Buisson (1998) *Care of Elderly People, Market Survey 1998*, Suffolk: Laing and Buisson.

Laing Buisson (2014) *Strategic Commissioning of Long-Term Care for Older People*, Suffolk: Laing and Buisson..

Laing Buisson (2018a) *Care of Elderly People: UK Market Survey 2017/18*, Suffolk: Laing and Buisson.

Laing Buisson (2018b) *UK Healthcare Market Review, 31st Edition*, Suffolk: Laing and Buisson.

Legal & General (2020) *The Isolation Economy*. Available at: https://www.legalandgeneralgroup.com/media/17802/lg_isolationeconomy_report_final-pages.pdf

Le Grand, J. (1991) Quasi-markets and social policy, *The Economic Journal*, 101(408): 1256–67.

Le Grand, J. (2009) *The Other Invisible Hand: Delivering Public Services through Choice and Competition*. Princeton: Princeton University Press.

Leibowitz, J. and Goodwin, T. (2018) *What Next for the Local Wealth Building Movement?*, Centre for Local Economic Strategies. Available at: https://cles.org.uk/blog/what-next-for-the-local-wealth-building-movement/

Lent, A. and Studdert, J. (2019) *The Community Paradigm: Why Public Services Need Radical Change and How It Can Be Achieved*, New Local Government Network. Available at: https://www.newlocal.org.uk/wp-content/uploads/2019/03/The-Community-Paradigm_New-Local.pdf

Lobao, L., Gray, M., Cox, K. and Kitson, M. (2018) The shrinking state? Understanding the assault on the public sector, *Cambridge Journal of Regions, Economy and Society*, 11(3): 389–408.

Localgiving (2018) *Local Charity and Community Group Sustainability Report 2017/18*. Available at: https://localgiving.org/about/reports/local-charity-and-community-group1718

Local Government Act (1985) London: The Stationery Office. Available at: https://www.legislation.gov.uk/ukpga/1985/51/contents

Local Government and Social Care Ombudsman (2019a) *Review of Adult Social Care Complaints 2018–19*. Available at: https://www.lgo.org.uk/information-centre/reports/annual-review-reports/adult-social-care-reviews

Local Government and Social Care Ombudsman (2019b) *Caring about Complaints.* Available at: https://www.lgo.org.uk/information-centre/reports/focus-reports

Local Government Association (2017) *Encouraging Innovation in Local Government Procurement Report.* Available at: https://www.local.gov.uk/sites/default/files/documents/4.35%20Encouraging%20Innovation%20in%20LG%20Procurement_v04_0.pdf

Local Government Association (2020a) *Rethinking Local.* Available at: https://www.local.gov.uk/sites/default/files/documents/3.70%20Rethinking%20local_%23councilscan_landscape_FINAL.pdf

Local Government Association (2020b) *Adult Social Care: Seven Principles for Reform.* Available at: https://local.gov.uk/adult-social-care-seven-principles-reform

Local Government Association (2020c) *The Lives We Want To Lead.* Available at: https://local.gov.uk/sites/default/files/documents/Adult-social-care-green-paper-full-research-report-final.pdf

Localism Act (2011) London: The Stationery Office. Available at: https://www.legislation.gov.uk/ukpga/2011/20/contents/enacted

Loney, M. (1981) The British community development projects: questioning the state, *Community Development Journal*, 16(1): 55–66.

Lukes, S. (2005) *Power: A Radical View*, London: Palgrave Macmillan.

Lyons Inquiry (2007) *Place-Shaping: A Shared Ambition for the Future of Local Government.* Available at: https://assets.publishing.service.gov.uk/government/uploads/system/uploads/attachment_data/file/229035/9780119898552.pdf

Malnutrition Task Force (2020) *State of the Nation: Older People and Malnutrition in the UK Today.* Available at: https://www.malnutritiontaskforce.org.uk/sites/default/files/2019-09/State%20of%20the%20Nation.pdf

Mannion, R. (2014) Enabling compassionate healthcare: perils, prospects and perspectives, *International Journal of Health Policy Management*, 2(3): 115–17.

Marshall, T.H. (1950) *Citizenship and Social Class*, Cambridge: Cambridge University Press.

Martinez, C. and Pritchard, J. (2019) *Proceed with Caution: What Makes Personal Budgets Work?*, Reform. Available at: https://reform.uk/sites/default/files/2019-02/Personal%20Budgets_AW_4_0.pdf

Mayer, J. and Timms, N. (1970) *The Client Speaks,* London: Routledge and Kegan Paul.

McBride, J. and Smith, A. (2018) *The Forgotten Workers Report*, University of Durham. Available at: https://www.dur.ac.uk/resources/business/research/235099ForgottenWorkersBooklet.pdf

McCafferty, S., Williams, I. and Hunter, D. (2012) NHS world class commissioning – competencies, *Journal of Health Services Research and Policy*, 17: 40–8.

McConnell, A. (2015) What is policy failure? A primer to help navigate the maze, *Public Policy and Administration*, 30(3/4): 221–42.

McGough, L. and Swinney, P. (2015) *Mapping Britain's Public Finances Where is Tax Raised, and Where is it Spent?*, Centre for Cities. Available at: https://www.centreforcities.org/wp-content/uploads/2015/07/15-07-06-Mapping-Britains-Public-Finances.pdf

McLaughlin, H. (2009) What's in a name: 'client', 'patient', 'customer', 'consumer', 'expert by experience', 'service user' – what's next?, *British Journal of Social Work*, 39(6): 1101–17.

Means, R., Morbey, H. and Smith, R. (2002) *From Community Care to Market Care? The Development of Welfare Services for Older People*, Bristol: Policy Press.

Mental Health Act (1983) London: The Stationery Office. Available at: https://www.legislation.gov.uk/ukpga/1983/20/contents

Migration Advisory Committee (2018) *EEA Migration in the UK: Final Report*, London. Available at: https://assets.publishing.service.gov.uk/government/uploads/system/uploads/attachment_data/file/741926/Final_EEA_report.PDF

Miller, E. and Gwynne, G. (1972) *A Life Apart*, London: Tavistock.

Ministry of Housing and Local Government (1967) *Management of Local Government*. London: HMSO.

Mintrom, M. (2010) Public policy: why ethics matters, in J. Boston, A. Bradstock and D. Eng (eds) *Public Policy: Why Ethics Matters*, Canberra: Australian National University.

Moriarty, J. (2017) Business ethics, in *The Stanford Encyclopaedia of Philosophy*. Available at: https://plato.stanford.edu/entries/ethics-business/

National Audit Office (2011) *Oversight of User Choice and Provider Competition on Care Markets*. Available at: https://www.nao.org.uk/wp-content/uploads/2011/09/10121458.pdf

National Audit Office (2013) *Over-optimism in Government Projects*. Available at: https://www.nao.org.uk/wp-content/uploads/2013/12/10320-001-Over-optimism-in-government-projects.pdf

National Audit Office (2016) *Personalised Commissioning in Adult Social Care*. Available at: https://www.nao.org.uk/wp-content/uploads/2016/03/Personalised-commissioning-in-adult-social-care-update.pdf

National Audit Office (2018a) *Financial Sustainability of Local Authorities*. Available at: https://www.nao.org.uk/wp-content/uploads/2018/03/Financial-sustainabilty-of-local-authorites-2018.pdf

National Audit Office (2018b) *Developing New Models of Care through NHS Vanguards*. Available at: https://www.nao.org.uk/wp-content/uploads/2018/06/Developing-new-care-models-through-NHS-Vanguards.pdf

National Audit Office (2018c) *The Adult Social Care Workforce in England*, London. Available at: https://www.nao.org.uk/wp-content/uploads/2018/02/The-adult-social-care-workforce-in-England.pdf

National Audit Office (2019) *Transforming Rehabilitation: Progress Review*. Available at: https://www.nao.org.uk/wp-content/uploads/2019/02/Transforming-Rehabilitation-Progress-review.pdf

National Audit Office (2020a) *Overview of the UK Government's Response to the COVID-19 Pandemic*. Available at: https://www.nao.org.uk/wp-content/uploads/2020/05/Overview-of-the-UK-governments-response-to-the-COVID-19-pandemic.pdf

National Audit Office (2020b) *Readying the NHS and Adult Social Care in England for COVID-19*. Available at: https://www.nao.org.uk/wp-content/uploads/2020/06/Readying-the-NHS-and-adult-social-care-in-England-for-COVID-19.pdf

National Audit Office (2020c) *Local Authority Investment in Commercial Property*. Available at: https://www.nao.org.uk/wp-content/uploads/2020/02/Local-authority-investment-in-commercial-property.pdf

Naylor A (2020) *Unforgotten: The People, Lost and Found, in Receipt of Social Care*, Future Care Capital, Social Care Data Finder. Available at: https://futurecarecapital.org.uk/latest/social-care-data-finder/

Naylor, C. and Wellings, D. (2019) *A Different Approach to Health and Care: Lessons from the Wigan Deal*, London: King's Fund. Available at: https://www.kingsfund.org.uk/sites/default/files/2019-07/A%20citizen-led%20report%20final%20%2819.6.19%29.pdf

NCVO (National Council for Voluntary Organisations) (2019) *The Civil Society Almanac, 2019*. Available at: https://data.ncvo.org.uk/

NDTI (National Development Team for Inclusion) (2020) *Community Led Support Evidence and Learning Briefings 2020*. Available at: https://www.ndti.org.uk/assets/files/CLS_Paper_1_Findings_MAY_2020_Fnl.pdf

Needham, C. (2014) *Micro-enterprises: Small Enough to Care?*, University of Birmingham. Available at: https://www.birmingham.ac.uk/Documents/college-social-sciences/social-policy/HSMC/research/micro-enterprise/Micro-enterprise-full-report,-final.pdf

Needham, C. (2018) Best of both worlds, *International Journal of Health Policy and Management*, 7(4): 356–8.

Needham, C. and Carr, S. (2009) *Co-production: An Emerging Evidence Base for Adult Social Care Transformation*, Social care Institute for Excellence. Available at: https://www.scie.org.uk/publications/briefings/briefing31/

Needham, C., Hall, K., Allen, K., Burn, E., Mangan, C. and Henwood, M. (2018) *Market Shaping and Personalisation in Social Care: A Realist Synthesis of the Literature*, Health Services Management Centre, University of Birmingham. Available at: https://www.birmingham.ac.uk/Documents/college-social-sciences/social-policy/HSMC/research/market-shaping-and-personalisation-social-care.pdf

Needham, C., Allen, K., Burn, E., Hall, K., Mangan, C., Al-Janabi, H., Tahir, W., Carr S., Glasby, J., Henwood, M., McKay, S. and Brant, I. (2020) *Shifting Shapes*, University of Birmingham. Available at: https://research.birmingham.ac.uk/portal/files/106824127/Shifting_Shapes_final_report_Oct_2020.pdf

Nesta and SCIE (Social Care Institute for Excellence) (2019) *Growing Innovative Models of Health, Care and Support for Adults*. Available at: https://www.scie.org.uk/future-of-care/adults

Newcastle Council for Voluntary Service (2018) *Do We Need to Talk? Public Sector Procurement and Contracts*. Available at: https://www.bl.uk/collection-items/do-we-need-to-talk-public-sector-procurement-and-contracts-a-thought-piece#

New Economics Foundation (2019) *Rating Retention: Options for Redesigning the Business Rates Retention System*. Available at: https://neweconomics.org/uploads/files/Rating-Retention.pdf

New Local Government Network (2018) *From Transactions to Changemaking: Rethinking Partnerships between the Public and Private Sectors*. Available at: https://www.basw.co.uk/system/files/resources/From-Transactions-to-Changemaking-1.pdf

NHS Digital (2019a) *Personal Social Services Survey of Adult Carers in England 2018-19*. Available at: https://digital.nhs.uk/data-and-information/publications/statistical/personal-social-services-survey-of-adult-carers/england-2018-19

NHS Digital (2019b) *Adult Social Care Activity and Finance Report, England 2018–19*. Available at: https://digital.nhs.uk/data-and-information/publications/statistical/adult-social-care-activity-and-finance-report/2019-20

NHS England (2019a) *Universal Personalised Care: Implementing the Comprehensive Model*. Available at: https://www.england.nhs.uk/wp-content/uploads/2019/01/universal-personalised-care.pdf

NHS England (2019b) *NHS Long-Term Plan*. Available at: https://www.longtermplan.nhs.uk/

NHS Support Federation (2017) *Time to End the NHS Experiment with the Market?*. Available at: https://www.nhsforsale.info/privatisation-report-december-2017/

Office for Disability Issues (2008) *Independent Living: A Cross-Government Strategy about Independent Living for Disabled People*. Available at: https://www.bl.uk/collection-items/independent-living-a-crossgovernment-strategy-about-independent-living-for-disabled-people

Office for National Statistics (2020a) *Labour Market Overview, UK: June 2020*. Available at: https://www.ons.gov.uk/employmentandlabourmarket/peopleinwork/employmentandemployeetypes/bulletins/uklabourmarket/june2020

Office for National Statistics (2020b) *Social Capital in the UK: 2020*. Available at: https://www.ons.gov.uk/peoplepopulationandcommunity/wellbeing/bulletins/socialcapitalintheuk/2020

Office for National Statistics (2020c) *Impact of Coronavirus in Care Homes in England*. Available at: https://www.ons.gov.uk/peoplepopulationandcommunity/healthandsocialcare/conditionsanddiseases/articles/impactofcoronavirusincarehomesinenglandvivaldi/26mayto19june2020

Onward (2020) *The State of our Social Fabric*. Available at: https://www.ukonward.com/wp-content/uploads/2020/09/The-State-of-our-Social-Fabric.pdf

Osborne, D. and Gaebler, T. (1992) *Reinventing Government*, Boston: Addison-Wesley Publication Company.

Parker, J. (1965) *Local Health and Welfare Services*, London: Allen and Unwin.

Parker, S. (2015) *Taking Power Back: Putting People in Charge of Politics*, Bristol: Policy Press.

Peckham, S., Hudson, B., Hunter, D.J., Redgate, S. and White, G. (2020) *Improving Choices for Care: A Strategic Research Initiative on the Implementation of the Care Act 2014*, National Institute for Health Research.

Phillips, D. and Simpson, P. (2018) *Changes in Councils Adult Social Care and Overall Spending in England, 2009–10 to 2017–18*, London: Institute for Fiscal Studies. Available at: https://www.ifs.org.uk/uploads/BN240.pdf

Pierson, J. (2008) *Going Local: Working in Communities and Neighbourhoods*, London: Routledge.

Pierson, P. (1994) *Dismantling the Welfare State*, Cambridge: Cambridge University Press.

Political Studies Association (2016) *Towards a New Deal for Care and Carers: Report of the Commission on Care*, London. Available at: http://www.commissiononcare.org/wp-content/uploads/2016/10/Web-Care-Comission-Towards-a-new-deal-for-care-and-carers-v1.0.pdf

Prime Minister's Strategy Unit (2005) *Improving the Life Chances of Disabled People*. Available at: https://www.basw.co.uk/system/files/resources/basw_113152-3_0.pdf

Pritchard, J. and Lasko-Skinner, R. (2019) *Please Procure Responsibly: The State of Public Service Commissioning*, London: Reform.

Propper, C., Stockton, I. and Stoye, G. (2020) *Covid-19 and the Disruptions to the Health and Social Care of Older People in England*, Institute for Fiscal Studies. Available at: https://ifs.org.uk/uploads/BN309-COVID-19-and-disruptions-to-the-health-and-social-care-of-older-people-in-England-1.pdf

Public Services (Social Value) Act (2012) London: The Stationery Office. Available at: https://www.legislation.gov.uk/ukpga/2012/3/enacted

Rachels, J. and Rachels, S. (2015) *The Elements of Moral Philosophy* (8th edn), New York, NY: McGraw-Hill.

Rahman, F. (2018) *The Generation of Poverty: Poverty Over the Life Course for Different Generations*, London: Resolution Foundation. Available at: https://www.resolutionfoundation.org/app/uploads/2019/05/Generation-of-Poverty-Report.pdf

Rawls, J. (1971) *A Theory of Justice*, Cambridge, MA: Belknap Press.

Redcliffe-Maud Commission (1969) *Royal Commission on Local Government in England* (vol 1). London: HMSO.

Rees, S., Sophocleous, C. and Hirst, N. (2017) *Delivering Transformation in Wales: Social Services and Wellbeing (Wales) Act 2014: Interim Findings*, Cardiff: Wales Institute of Social and Economic Research. Available at: https://wiserd.ac.uk/sites/default/files/documents/eng_sswba_briefingpaper_wcc_final_27.11.17_1.pdf

Resolution Foundation (2018) *Healthy Finances? Options for Funding an NHS Spending Increase.* Available at: https://www.resolutionfoundation.org/app/uploads/2018/06/Healthy-Finances.pdf

Roberts, C., Blakely, G. and Murphy, L. (2019) *A Wealth of Difference: Reforming the Taxation of Wealth,* London: IPPR. Available at: https://www.ippr.org/files/2018-10/cej-a-wealth-of-difference-sept18.pdf

Rome, A. (2020) *Profit Making and Risk in Independent Children's Social Care Placement Providers,* Exeter: Revolution Consulting. Available at: https://www.revolution-consulting.org/wp-content/uploads/2020/03/Profit-Making-and-Risk-in-Independent-Childrens-Social-Care-Placement-Providers-Final-29-Feb-2020-report.pdf

Ruano, J. and Profirolu, M. (2019) *The Palgrave Handbook of Decentralisation in Europe,* London: Palgrave Handbooks.

Rubery, J., Grimshaw, D., Hebson, G. and Ugarte, S. (2015) Time as contested terrain in the management and experience of domiciliary care work in England, *Human Resource Management in Health Care and Elderly Care,* September/October: 753-772. Available at: https://onlinelibrary.wiley.com/doi/abs/10.1002/hrm.21685

Rummery, K. and Glendinning, C. (2000) *Primary Care and Social Services: Developing New Partnerships for Older People,* Abingdon: Radcliffe.

Ryan, F. (2019) *Crippled: Austerity and the Demonization of Disabled People,* Brooklyn: Verso.

Sandel, M. (2012) *What Money Can't Buy: The Moral Limits of Markets,* London: Allen Lane.

Sanford, M. (2019a) Is devolution to England's cities here to stay?, in Institute for Government (ed) *Has Devolution Worked?,* London: Institute for Government. Available at: https://www.instituteforgovernment.org.uk/sites/default/files/publications/has-devolution-worked-essay-collection-FINAL.pdf

Sanford, M. (2019b) Where do you draw the line? Local administrative boundaries in England, House of Commons Library Briefing Paper. Available at: https://commonslibrary.parliament.uk/research-briefings/cbp-8619/

Sasse, T., Britchfield, C. and Davies, N. (2020) *Carillion: Two Years On,* London: Institute for Government. Available at: https://www.instituteforgovernment.org.uk/sites/default/files/publications/carillion-two-years-on.pdf

Seebohm Committee (1968) *Report of the Committee on Local Authority and Allied Personal Social Services,* London: HMSO.

Scourfield, P. (2012) Caretelization revisited and the lessons of Southern Cross, *Critical Social Policy,* 32 (1): 137-148. Available at: https://doi.org/10.1177/0261018311425202

Sharpe, L.J. (1965) *Why Local Democracy?,* London: Fabian Society.

Simpkin, M. (1979) *Trapped within Welfare,* London: Macmillan.

Skelcher, C. (2000) Changing images of the State: overloaded, hollowed-out, congested, *Public Policy and Administration,* 15(3): 3-19. Available at: https://journals.sagepub.com/doi/pdf/10.1177/095207670001500302

Skills for Care (2018a) *The State of the Adult Social Care Sector and Workforce in England,* London. Available at: https://www.skillsforcare.org.uk/adult-social-care-workforce-data/Workforce-intelligence/publications/national-information/The-state-of-the-adult-social-care-sector-and-workforce-in-England.aspx

Skills for Care (2018b) *Social Work Education,* London. Available at: https://www.skillsforcare.org.uk/adult-social-care-workforce-data/Workforce-intelligence/documents/Social-Work-Education-in-England.pdf

Skills for Care (2018c) *The Economic Value of the Adult Social Care Sector.* Available at: https://www.skillsforcare.org.uk/Documents/About/sfcd/Economic-value-of-the-adult-social-care-sector-UK.pdf

Skills for Care (2019) *The Size and Structure of the Adult Social Care Sector and Workforce in England.* Available at: https://www.skillsforcare.org.uk/adult-social-care-workforce-data/Workforce-intelligence/documents/Size-of-the-adult-social-care-sector/Size-and-Structure-2020.pdf

Slasberg, C., Beresford, P. and Schofield, P. (2015) Further lessons from the continuing failure of the national strategy to deliver personal budgets and personalisation, *Research, Policy and Planning,* 31(1): 43–53.

Smith, R. (2019) How health care is eating other public services, *British Medical Journal,* 4 December.

Smith, R., Lloyd, L., Cameron, A., Johnson, E. and Willis, P. (2019) What is (adult) social care in England? Its origins and meaning, *Research, Policy and Planning,* 33(2): 45–56.

Social Care Futures (2019) *Talking about a Brighter Social Care Future.* Available at: https://socialcarefuture.files.wordpress.com/2019/10/ic-scf-report-2019-h-web-final-111119.pdf

Social Enterprise (2016) *Procuring for Good: How the Social Value Act is Being Used by Local Authorities,* London. Available at: https://www.socialenterprise.org.uk/wp-content/uploads/2019/05/Procuring_for_Good_FINAL.pdf

Social Science Research Unit (2012) *Commissioning in Health, Education and Social Care*, London: University of London. Available at: https://eppi.ioe.ac.uk/cms/Portals/0/PDF%20reviews%20and%20summaries/Commissioning%202012Newman.pdf?ver=2012-09-17-123424-943

Spiers, G., Matthews, F., Moffatt, S., Barker, R., Jarvis, H., Stow, D., Kingston, A. and Hanratty, B. (2019) Does older adults' use of social care influence their healthcare utilisation? A systematic review of international evidence, *Health and Social Care in the Community*, 27(5): 651–62.

Stewart, J. (2014) An era of continuing change: reflections on local government in England, 1974–2014, *Local Government Studies*, 40(6): 835–50.

Sturgess, G. (2018) Public service commissioning: origins, influences and characteristics, *Policy Design and Practice*, 1(3): 155–68.

Sutherland Report (1999) *With Respect to Old Age: Long Term Care – Rights and Responsibilities: A Report by the Royal Commission on Long Term Care,* London: The Stationery Office. Available at: https://webarchive.nationalarchives.gov.uk/20131205101144/http://www.archive.official-documents.co.uk/document/cm41/4192/4192.htm

Taylor, M., Langan, J. and Hoggett, P. (1995) *Encouraging Diversity: Voluntary and Private Organisations in Community Care*, Aldershot: Arena.

Thane, P. (1996) *Foundations of the Welfare State*, London: Longman.

Think Local Act Personal (2018) *Beyond Direct Payments*. Available at: https://www.thinklocalactpersonal.org.uk/_assets/News/BeyondDirectPayments.pdf

Thoburn, J. (2017) In defence of a university social work education, *Journal of Children's Services*, 12(2/3): 97–106.

Thomas, C. and Quilter-Pinner, H. (2020) *Care Fit For Carers*, Institute for Public Policy Research. Available at: https://www.ippr.org/files/2020-04/1587632465_care-fit-for-carers-april20.pdf

Thompson, G., Frances, J., Levacic, R. and Mitchell, J. (1994) *Markets, Hierarchies and Networks: The Coordination of Social Life*, London: Sage.

Timmins, N. (1995) *The Five Giants: A Biography of the Welfare State*, London: Harper Collins.

Tiratelli, L. and Kaye, S. (2020) *Communities and Coronavirus: The Rise of Mutual Aid,* London: New Local Government Network. Available at: https://www.newlocal.org.uk/wp-content/uploads/Communities-Vs-Corona-Virus-The-Rise-of-Mutual-Aid.pdf

Titmuss, R. (1997 [1970]) *The Gift Relationship: From Human Blood to Social Policy* (reprinted by the New Press with new chapters, eds John Ashton and Ann Oakley), London: LSE Books.

Townsend, P. (1964) *The Last Refuge. a Survey of Residential Institutions and Homes for the Aged in England and Wales*, London: Routledge & Kegan Paul.

Toynbee, P. and Walker, D. (2020) *The Lost Decade, 2010–2020*, London: Guardian Books.

Trade Union Council (2019) *General Council Report 2019*, London: Trade Union Congress. Available at: https://www.tuc.org.uk/sites/default/files/2019-08/General_Council_Report_2019_TUC_1.pdf

Tronto, J. (2010) Creating caring institutions: politics, plurality and purpose, *Ethics and Social Welfare*, 4(2): 158–71.

Tunstill, J. (2019) Pruned, policed and privatised: the knowledge base for children and families social work in England and Wales in 2019, *Social Work & Social Sciences Review*, 20(2): 57–76.

Tussell (2020) *Social Value Procurement: Local Authority League Tables*. Available at: https://www.tussell.com/insights/how-good-are-local-authorities-at-awarding-contracts-to-smes-and-vcses

Twigg, J. (1997) Bathing and the politics of care, *Social Policy & Administration*, 31(1): 61–72.

UK2070 Commission (2020) *Make No Little Plans: Acting at Scale for a Fairer and Stronger Future*. Available at: http://uk2070.org.uk/wp-content/uploads/2020/02/UK2070-FINAL-REPORT.pdf

Unison (2017a) *Unison's Ethical Care Charter*, London. Available at: https://www.unison.org.uk/content/uploads/2017/06/ethicalcarecharterEDITFINAL.pdf

Unison (2017b) *Home Care Survey 2017*, London. Available at: https://www.unison.org.uk/content/uploads/2017/09/UNISON-home-care-survey-2017.pdf

United Kingdom Home Care Association (2016) *An Overview of the Domiciliary Care Market in the United Kingdom*. Available at: https://www.ukhca.co.uk/downloads.aspx?ID=611

Unwin Inquiry (2018) *Civil Society Futures: The Story of Our Times*. Available at: https://civilsocietyfutures.org/final-reports/

Unwin, J. (2018) *Kindness, Emotions and Human Relationships: The Blind Spot in Public Policy*, Carnegie Trust. Available at: https://d1ssu070pg2v9i.cloudfront.net/pex/carnegie_uk_trust/2018/11/13152200/LOW-RES-3729-Kindness-Public-Policy3.pdf

Visram, S., Hunter, D., Perkins, N., Adams, L., Finn, R., Gosling, J. and Forrest, A. (2020) Health and wellbeing boards as theatres of accountability: a dramaturgical analysis, *Local Government Studies* (September). Available at: https://www.tandfonline.com/doi/full/10.1080/03003930.2020.1816543?scroll=top&needAccess=true

Walker, D. and Tizard, J. (2018) *Out of Control*, London: Smith Institute. Available at: http://www.smith-institute.org.uk/wp-content/uploads/2018/01/Out-of-contract-Time-to-move-on-from-the-%E2%80%98love-in%E2%80%99-with-outsourcing-and-PFI.pdf

Welsh Government (2015) *Well-Being of Future Generations Act*. Available at: https://www.futuregenerations.wales/about-us/future-generations-act/

Wenzel, L., Bennett, L., Bottery, S., Murray, L. and Sahib, B. (2018) *Approaches to Social Care Funding Options*, King's Fund. Available at: https://www.health.org.uk/publications/approaches-to-social-care-funding

We Own It (2019) *When We Own It: A Model for Public Ownership in the 21st Century*. Available at: https://weownit.org.uk/sites/default/files/attachments/When%20We%20Own%20It%20-%20A%20model%20for%20public%20ownership%20in%20the%2021st%20century.pdf

West, K. (2013) The grip of personalisation on adult social care: between managerial domination and fantasy, *Critical Social Policy*, 33(4): 638–57.

Williams, B. (2005) *In the Beginning Was the Deed*, Princeton: Princeton University Press.

Wilson, S., Davison, N., Clarke, C. and Casebourne, J. (2017) *Joining Up Public Services Around Local Citizen Needs*, London: Institute for Government.

Wistow, G. (2012) Still a fine mess? Local government and the NHS 1962 to 2012, *Journal of Integrated Care*, 20(2): 101–14.

Wistow, G., Knapp, M., Hardy, B. and Allen, C. (1994) *Social Care in a Mixed Economy*, Buckingham: Open University Press.

Wistow, G., Knapp, M., Hardy, B., Forder, J., Kendall, J. and Manning, R. (1996) *Social Care Markets: Progress and Prospects*, Buckingham: Open University Press.

Wootton, B. (1959) *Social Science and Social Pathology*, London: George Allen & Unwin.

Younghusband, E. (ed) (1965) *Social Work with Families, Readings in Social Work*, London: NISW and George Allen and Unwin.

Index

Note: Page numbers for tables appear in *italics*.

A

abuse 60–1, 100
accountability 128, 138
achievement, and well-being 109
Action Plan (Department of Health and
    Social Care) 127–8, 131, 132
administration, deficiencies in 118–19
administrative capacity 83–8, 89
affluent areas 49, 66
age discrimination 129–31
ageing, representations of 143
agencies 18, 20, 120
agenda 145–6
Age UK 43, 79
All-Party Parliamentary Group on
    Social Care 98
All-Party Parliamentary Group on
    Social Integration 123
All-Party Parliamentary Group on
    Wellbeing Economics 104
American Nursing Home Transparency
    and Improvement Act 2009 100
'anchor' institutions 109
anti-poverty practice 93
appeals process over denial of access to
    care 67
apprenticeship 99
asset-based working 108
Association for Public Service
    Excellence 110
Association of Directors of Adult Social
    Services (ADASS) 51, 77, 119
asylums 8
'asymmetrical' contracts 136
attachment 109
Audit Commission 18, 29, 140
austerity 42–4, 45, 50, 103, 112
Australia 135
Australian National Integrity
    Commission 135
autonomy 105, 109
availability 47–9

B

Bailey, R. 13
Baird et al 36
Banks, S. 91
Barchester 53

Barclay, Sir Peter 20
Barclay Report 20–1
Barnsley 109
basic co-production 106
Baxter et al 41–2
Bedford, S. 110–11
behaviour and incentives 137
Better Care Fund 76
Bevan, Nye 138
Big Society 88
Birmingham University 109
Blair government 88
blood donation 136–7
Brake, M. 13
Brexit 59, 97
British Academy 95
British Association of Social
    Workers 93, 101
British Council of Organisations of
    Disabled People 13
Broadhurst, S. 71
Brown, L. 11
Brown et al 109
budgets, personal 14, 38–9, 42, 45
building work, tendering 15
Burn, E. 43
business ethics 94
business rates 76, 78, 118
Business Rates Retention Scheme 76
Button, D. 110–11
The Buurtzorg model 108

C

care, ethics of 92
Care Act 2014 36, 38, 44, 57, 100–1,
    111, 142
    and COVID-19 125
    and Dilnot Report 80–1
    and eligibility criteria 49
    on financial oversight role 69
    Implementation Support
        Programme 141
    and market-shaping role on local
        authorities 33, 70, 71, 72
    and national minimum eligibility
        threshold 78
Care Certificate 97, 100
care charter 99
career progression 54–6, 98

care homes 16–18, 20, 27, 33, 47–8, 52–3
and agency staff 120
closures 50
cost 40
and COVID-19 121, 127, 129–30, 131
and large providers 104–5
quality of care 60
and regulation of managers 98
where income goes 100
Care Home Transparency Act 100
care management 21
care providers 27, 39, 40, 43, 110, 118
and Covid-19 121
and finances 69
Care Providers Alliance 121
Care Quality Commission 37, 51, 58, 61, 70, 99–100
and commissioning 114
and Coronavirus Act 2020 126
and Covid-19 deaths 127, 130
financial oversight role 69
and improvement support 140
on smaller facilities 105
Carers UK 44
Care Services Improvement Partnership 140
Carey, M. 21
Carey et al 28
Carillion 31–2, 63, 134
Carr, S. 39, 106
Case Con 13
case management 21
caseworker 12
Cavendish Review 55
central government 57, 77, 78, 83, 84, 85–6, 89
funded community development projects 13
no national budget for social care 75–6
centralised approach, outsourcing 32
Centre for Local Economic Strategies 102
Centre for Local Economic Studies 109
Certificate of Fundamental Care 55
challenge and accountability 138
Change Agent Team 140
charities 49, 105, 122
Charity Commission 36
Charity Organisation Society 12
check-in and chat volunteers 123
CHPI (Centre for Health and the Public Interest) 27, 52, 53, 65, 100
Chronically Sick and Disabled Persons Act 1970 7
citizenship 41, 139

civic life 77
civic participation 106
civil rights 139
civil society 49, 105
Civil Society Strategy 102
client–professional relationship 12
closed-door culture 32
Coalition government 2, 85, 88, 140
Code of Practice on Ethical Employment in Supply Chains 99
collective bargaining 56–7, 96–7
coloniser chains 27
commercial confidentiality 32
commissioning 31, 32–45, 94–115, 134, 146
Commissioning Academy 113
Commission on Economic Justice 95
Commission on Evidence-Based Policymaking (US) 135
Commission on the Funding of Care and Support 2
Committee on Standards in Public Life (CSPL) 133–4, 135
Commons Digital, Culture, Media and Sports Committee 122
Communities and Local Government, Department for 84–5
community 20–1, 105–6, 128
community businesses 108
Community Care (Direct Payments) Act 1996 13, 38, 106
Community Catalysts 107–8
community development 20, 24
community development projects (CDPs) 13
community engagement 21
community enterprises 106–7, 108
community ownership 109
the community paradigm 114
community response volunteers 123
community sector organisations 36, 49
community services 8–9, 18
community social services 49
community social work 20, 21
Companies Act 95
company law 95
competence, and ethical behaviour 92
competition 11, 23, 55, 67, 105, 120, 146
Competition and Markets Authority 33, 41, 52, 53, 67
complaints handling 67–8
complexity, and policymaking 137
compulsory competitive tendering 15
concern, and an ethical life 92
Conservative governments 2–3, 8, 11–12, 14, 15–16, 19
Conservative Party 2, 3

consolidated market 22–5, 29–30
construction and property groups 27
consumer citizens 139
consumer information 67, 72
consumerism 5, 41
consumer protection 67, 72
consumers 11
consumer sovereignty 146
continual professional
    development 99–100
continuing health care (CHC)
    assessments 126, 129
contracting 35
contracts 32
contract scoring systems 102
cooperative care transitions 110
Co-operative Development
    Scotland 110
Cooper et al 60–1
co-production 106, 109
Coronavirus (Scotland) (No.2) Act
    2020 126
Coronavirus Act 2020 124, 125–6
Coronavirus Business Interruption Loan
    Scheme 122
Coronavirus Job Retention
    Scheme 122
corporation tax 82
Corrigan, P. 13
cost-effectiveness 32
costs 17–18, 29, 36, 42, 52, 53, 136
    contributions towards 41, 79, 80
    and Covid-19 119, 121
    of renationalisation 64
    of residential care 40, 107
    savings by councils 33
    staff 54, 56, 60, 96, 118
    and Sutherland Report 82, 139
council-funded care home
    provision 17–18, 29
councils 16, 33, 67, 76–8, 85, 129, 132
    see also local authorities
council tax 43, 76, 77, 78
council tenants 15
counselling role of social work 20
county councils 19
COVID-19 76, 78, 100, 106, 117–32
crime 106
CSI Market Intelligence 47–8
Cumbers, A. 64
the 'customer,' strengthening 67–8, 72

D

Davies et al 34–5, 36
day services 19
deaths, due to COVID-19 127,
    129, 130

death tax 2
debt repayments 52
Delivery Board 141
dementia tax 2
deprived areas 43, 49, 76, 77–8
devolution 84
DHSS (Department of Health and
    Social Security) 49
diffusion 142
dignity 100, 107
Dilnot Report 80–1
directors' remuneration 52
Directory of Social Change 122
direct payments 13, 14, 37, 38–9, 45,
    71, 106
disability 3–4
    social model of 13
disabled people 12–13, 38, 39,
    101, 106
    and the Chronically Sick and Disabled
        Persons Act 7
    and COVID-19 130
    and personal budgets 45
disabled people's movement 13–14
disabled people's organisations
    (DPOs) 106
discourses 142, *143*
district councils 118
district nurses 108
distrust 106
domiciliary care 17, 27, 29, 48, 65,
    105, 108
    and 1989 White Paper 19
    and means test 79
    and 'task and time' model 60
    and zero-hours contracts 55

E

education 56, 101
elderly people 107–8, 123
    see also older people
eligibility criteria 22, 29, 42, 49,
    78, 145
emergent market 16–18, 28–9
emotion 92, 93
employee buy-outs 110
employment practice, ethical 94–100
employment rates, female 44
enabling role 24–5
England, lack of regulation of social
    care workforce unlike rest of
    UK 97–8
English Longitudinal Study of
    Ageing 44
enjoyment, and well-being 109
environmental health officers 120
established market 25–8, 30

estate levy 2
ethical behaviour 133–5
ethical employment practice 94–100
ethical framework for social care 128–9
ethical leadership 134
Ethical Leadership Commission 134–5
ethics 91–4, 99, 114, 115, 133
EU nationals 59
European Pillar of Social Rights 97
evidence-based policy 135, 137
Exercise Cygnus 130–1
expenditure
  buying goods and services from external suppliers 16
  reductions in 11, 54
  see also spending
experience good 41
exploitation 52–3

F

failure, policy 137–9
fatalism 43
female employment rates 44
female–male pay gap 54
financial assessment 16–17, 28–9
financial oversight 69
fit and proper person test 69–70
fixed-hours contract 97, 99
flexibility 24, 30, 37, 49, 107–8, 122, 128
Foundations for Evidence-Based Policymaking Act (US) 135
Four Seasons 51, 53
Fowler, Norman 15–16, 19
Fox, A. 39, 79, 105
fragility 50–1, 61, 66, 72, 117, 120–4
fragmentation 65–6, 72
free at the point of use 18, 29, 80, 82
Frontline 57
functional economic areas 85
funding 2, 20, 41, 75–83, 89, 117, 138
  of asylums 8
  due to COVID-19 118–19, 121–2, 132
  government to local councils 42, 43, 45
  and personal budgets 39
  of Seebohm model 10
  short-term 103
  start-up 104
  and the third sector 36
furloughing staff 122
Future Care Capital 61
Future Generations Commissioner 104
Future High Streets Fund 85

G

Gaebler, T. 28
Gamble, A. 84
geriatric hospital beds 18, 29
Germany 81, 82
The Gift Relationship (Titmuss) 136–7
'golden age' services 138
governance forum 110
governance framework 110
government funding, central 33, 42, 45, 75–6, 77, 78
  and community development projects 13
  and Skills for Care 57
grants 76
Greater London Council 19
Greater Manchester Combined Authority 102–3
Greater Manchester Local Commissioning Academy 114
Green, Damian 81
Green Paper, adult social care 2–3
Griffiths, James 138
Griffiths, Sir Roy 18–19, 29
Griffiths Report 18–19, 20, 29
Gwynne, G. 8

H

Hambleton, R. 84
Hanna, T. 64
Hardy, B. 17
Hare, R.M. 91
harm, minimising 128
Hayes et al 126, 127
HC-One 53, 121
health 3, 8, 100
Health, Department of 68–9
Health Advisory Service 140
Health and Care Professionals Council 97
Health and Safety Executive 126
Health and Social Care, Department of 57, 67, 87, 112, 125, 141
Health and Social Care Act 2012 126
health and social care budgets 112
health authorities 23
healthcare 82
  see also NHS
Health Education England 57
Health Foundation 82
Health Services and Public Health Act 1968 7
Held, V. 92
Henkel, M. 140
Henricson, C. 93
Henwood et al 41
herd immunity 129, 130

hierarchy 144, 145, 147
Hollis, Florence 12
home care 25, *26*, 66, 71
  and commissioning 34–5
  and COVID-19 121
  workers 60, 98
  and zero-hours contracts 120
Home Care Association 121
homes, selling to pay for care costs 41
Hospital Plan, 1962 8–9
hospitals
  delayed transfers of care from 86
  NHS long-stay 25
hotel and leisure interests 27
in-house delivery 109
household sector 27
House of Commons Health
  Committee 69
House of Commons Public Accounts
  Committee 54, 84–5, 111–12
housing assets 79, 82
Housing Reform Act 1988 15
Hudson, B. 86
Hunt, Jeremy 2–3
hypothecation 81–2

I

Immigration (EU Withdrawal) Bill 59
Implementation Support
  Programme 141
Improved Better Care Fund grant 76
improvement capability 140
improvement support 140–1
incentives 98, 118, 137
inclusiveness, and ethical
  framework 128
income-and asset-based means
  test 17, 28–9
income tax 82
Independent Age 67–8
independent living centre,
  Hampshire 106
Independent Living Movement 13
Independent Living Strategy 106
independent sector 17, 19, 25, 56
  see also private sector
Infection Control Fund 119
informal carers 44, 45
informal sector 27
innovation 142, 143
insecurity, workplace 55
Institute for Government 88
Institute for Public Policy Research
  (IPPR) 54
integrated care 87–8
Integrated Care Network 140
integrity 92

intermediate co-production 106
International Monetary Fund 10
International Year of Disabled People,
  1981 12–13
investment, lack of, in
  welfare institutions 8
IPPR (Institute for Public Policy
  Research) 56, 59, 95, 96, 97
Ireland, Northern 98
isolation 106, 107, 123
issue 145

J

Jacobs, L. 11
Japan 81
jobs, social care 1, 53–4, 58–9, 60, 108,
  113, 131
Johnson, Boris 3, 5, 141
Johnson et al 142
joined-up services 86–8
joint commissioning 33, 35, 86, *87*
Just Group 40

K

kindness 93, 136
King's Fund 51, 82
Klinenberg, E. 105
Knight et al 114
Kuhn, Thomas 144

L

Labour governments 2, 8, 10
labour market regulations 11, 98,
  99–100
Labour Party 2, 3, 22, 65
labour work, tendering 15
Landau, K. 71
The Language of Morals (Hare) 91
large providers 34, 50, 53, 70,
  94, 104–5
  able to expand 26, 30
  and leakage 52
leadership, ethical 134
leakage 52, 53
learning disabilities 3, 4, 8, 13, 70–
  1, 127
'left behind' areas 49
  see also deprived areas
legislation on care homes 100
Le Grand, J. 28
Lent, A. 114
Leonard, P. 13
life expectancy 1
living costs 82
living wage 54, 77, 96, 99
Living Wage Foundation 96
Local Area Coordination 107

local authorities 18–20, 21–5, 29–30, 65, 83–4
  and Care Act 2014 33, 36
  and care home beds 47–9
  and commissioning 31, 37, 95
  and COVID-19 funding 118–19
  and direct labour work 15
  and disabled people 106
  and easement of statutory duties 124–6
  and ethical framework 129
  and funded support 45
  and Living Wage Foundation 96
  and market position statements 34
  and market-shaping 70, 71–2, 111
  and National Assistance Act 7
  new powers to buy out providers 110
  and NHS 138
  residential care 17–18
  and Shared Lives 107
  and social services departments 9–10
  spending 4
  and well-being 101–2
Local Authority Social Services Act 1970 10, 14
local change 141
local councils 16, 85, 129
  see also local authorities
local enterprise partnerships (LEPs) 85
local government 50, 75–9, 85–6, 88, 89, 102
  see also local authorities
Local Government Act 1985 19
Local Government Act 1988 15
Local Government and Social Care Ombudsman 67
Local Government Association 42, 44, 100, 111
Localism Act 2011 88
local private companies 109
local relationships 106
local suppliers 109
local validation 142, 143
local wealth building 109
loneliness 107, 123
low pay 54–5, 56, 96, 100
low policy salience 117, 124–8
low status 55–8
Lukes, Steven 145
Lyons Inquiry 88

M

Major, John 133
male–female pay gap 54
malnutrition 44
Malnutrition Task Force 44
managed market 71, 72

management buyouts 23
management fees 52
Manchester 109
manipulation 145, 146
Mannion, R. 60
the market 16–30, 66–73, 135–7, 144, 145, 146
market-based paradigm 144
market failure 50, 61, 66, 68, 69
market fragility 50–1, 61, 66, 72, 117, 120–1
marketisation 4, 25
market model 16, 22, 30, 66, 72, 135, 138
  and collapse of Southern Cross 50
  and ethical model 114
  social care ill-suited to 25
  at tipping point 51
market oversight 68–9
market position statements 33–4
market regulation 29
market rights 139
market-shaping 11, 33, 43, 68, 69–72, 111
Marshall, TH 139
McConnell, A. 137
McLaughlin, H. 68
meal services 7
means test 14, 17, 22, 45, 79, 82
  and Dilnot Report 80
  and Royal Commission 2
mediating role 34
mental health 3, 8, 100
mental health hospitals 8–9
metro mayors 85
micro-commissioners 71
micro-enterprises 108
micro-providers 105, 106–7
Midlands Engine 85
migrant workers 59
Migration Advisory Committee 59
Miller, E. 8
minimum wage 54, 77, 96, 97, 100
Minstrom, M. 92
Monitor 69
moral agents 60, 91, 93, 115
morality 93
morals 136
Morris, Alf 7
Municipal Corporations Act 1835 83
municipal enterprises 109

N

narrow approach 32
National Assistance (Amendment) Act 1962 7
National Assistance Act 1948 7

National Audit Office 57, 58, 78, 85–6, 112, 137–8
National Care Service 2, 65
National Council for Voluntary Organisations 37
National Institute for Health and Clinical Excellence (NICE) 130
National Institute for Social Work 20
national insurance contributions 82
National Integrity Commission Bill (Australia) 135
National Living Wage 96, 118
national minimum eligibility threshold 78
national minimum wage 77
  see also minimum wage
National Resources Wales 103
national workforce strategy 57
need 12–13
Needham, C. 43, 105, 106
Needham et al 35, 36, 71
needs assessments 22, 82, 124–5
neglect 60, 100
neighbourhood groups 125
Neighbourhood Renewal 88
neighbourhoods 105
neoliberalism 11, 13–14, 15, 16, 39, 138
Netherlands 108
network development role 35
networks 144, 147
Newcastle Council for Voluntary Service 37
New Deal for Communities 88
New Homes Bonus 76
New Labour 14
New Local Government Network 32, 102
new localism 88
New Philanthropy Capital 49
new public management 15, 28, 29, 136
New Zealand 104
NHS 82, 83, 86, 126–7, 138
  and care workers 57
  and CHCs 126
  and COVID-19 129, 130
  funding 76, 78
  and geriatric hospital beds 18, 29
  long-stay hospitals 25
  and nurses in care homes 58
  and personal budgets 38
  and purchaser–provider split 15
  transport volunteers 123
  unhitching adult social care from 98
  and volunteering 123–4
  and workforce planning 57

NHS and Community Care Act 1990 19, 21–2
NHS England 87
NHS Funding Act 78
NHS Long-Term Plan 38, 111
NHS trusts 23
'NHS Volunteer' scheme 123
Nolan Principles 133–4
non-EU migrants 59
non-governmental organisations 28
non-residential support 17
non-statutory sector 20, 21, 28, 34
  see also private sector
Northamptonshire County Council 84
the North East 78
Northern Ireland 98
Northern Ireland Social Care Council 98
Northern Powerhouse 85
Northern Rock 64
not-for-profit companies 23, 25, 26, 30, 51–2, 61, 62
not-for-profit trusts 23
Nuffield Trust 88
nurses 58, 108
nursing, and care home beds 48
nursing homes 17, 29, 65, 100

O
Office of National Statistics 105
offshore ownership 52
older people 1, 3, 8, 43–4, 79, 107–8, 143
  and COVID-19 129
  financial assessment of 16–17, 28–9
  and personal budgets 39, 45
  and risk 81
open market 71, 72
Osborne, D. 28
Our Place 88
outsourcing 31–2, 63–4, 65, 68, 119–20
Outsourcing Playbook 134
overseeing role 34

P
pandemic, COVID-19 76, 78, 100, 106, 117–32
paradigm shift 144
partnership 71, 72
path dependency 138, 144
patient transport volunteers 123
pay 54–5, 56, 96–7, 98, 100
payments, direct 13, 14, 37, 38–9, 45, 71, 106
penetration, market 65

personal budgets 14, 38–9, 42, 45, 111, 112
personal care 39, 82, 107–8, 138–9
personal commissioning 41, 111–14
personal development 24
personal health budgets 111, 112
personalisation, commissioning 39, 71, *87*
personalised domiciliary care 105
personal social services 10
philanthropy 49, 83, 145
Phillips, D. 77–8
physical health 100
physically disabled people 13
'place' agenda *87*, 109
place-based commissioning 88
place-based neighbourhood working 108
Planning and Local Government Act 1980 15
policy failure 137–9
policy salience, low 117, 124–8
policy status 138
poor areas 76
  see also deprived areas
Poor Law 7
poverty 75, 93, 104
Powell, Enoch 8
power 145–7
Power to Change 107, 108
PPE (personal protective equipment) 127, 129–30
practical improvement support 140–1
Preston 109
prevention 43, *87*
primary care networks (PCNs) 88
Prime Minister's Strategy Unit 106
Principles of Commissioning and Wellbeing 113–14
private (for-profit) agencies 23
private care homes 16–18, 28–9
private for-profit healthcare groups 27
private for-profit providers 25
private not-for-profit healthcare groups 27
private providers 24, 27
private sector 25, 30, 49, 56, 61, 119–20
privatisation 20, 47, 54, 61–2, 66
procurement 31, 32, 35, 37, 71, 72, 114
  and ethical standards 134
  and social value strategy 101
Procurement Reform (Scotland) Act 2014 99
professional–client relationship 5, 12
professional regulation 55, 97–8
professional status 113

for-profit companies 25, 26, 30, 51, 54
profiteering 52–3
profit maximisation 24, 52
Programme Board 141
Programme Management Office 141
property costs 52
proportionality 128
provider options 23
public administration 83, 89
public choice theory 136
public companies 61, 62
public expenditure 11, 16, 54
Public Health England 130–1
public ownership model 4
public sector 11, 27, 56
Public Sector Transformation Academy 113
public service boards 103
public services 19, 136
Public Services (Social Value) Act 2012 101–2
Public Values Act 102
purchaser–provider split 15, 16, 32, 45, 86–7
pure market 80
Putting People First 112–13

Q

quality, job 99
quality monitoring 35
quality of care 58–61, 62, 105
quality of service 67
quasi-markets 4, 11, 15, 28, 37, 80
Quilter-Pinner, H. 131

R

radical social work 13, 14
Rawls, J. 82
reasonableness 128
recruitment 58, 59–60, 99, 103, 113, 123
Redcliffe-Maud Report 88
regional partnership boards (RPBs) 103
regional social value (RSV) forums 103
regulated market 18–22
regulation 11, 98, 99–100
renationalisation 64–5, 66, 72
residential care 8, 16–18, 25, *26*, 65, 79, 127
  see also care homes
residents, treating fairly 67
respect 91, 92, 128
respite services 19
responsibility, and moral competence in public life 92
resuscitation categorisation 130
revenue support grant 75, 76
risk 21, 29, 107, 134, 136, 137

and companies 95
and Covid-19 120, 122, 125
and old age 81
and primary care networks 88
social 82
risk aversion 43, 103, 104
Royal College of Care Work 99
Royal Commission, 1997 82
Royal Commission, 1999 2
Royal Commission on Long Term
    Care 10, 80, 139
Royal Voluntary Service 123
Ryan, E. 130

S

safety-net approach 20
sale and leaseback 52
Sandel, Michael 136, 137
Sanford, M. 85
Scotland 82, 96, 97–8, 126
Scottish Social Services Council 98
security
    of care 3
    of workforce 56, 65, 96, 97, 98
Seebohm Committee 9–10, 14
Seebohm model 14, 18, 29
Seebohm Report 20, 139
self-funders 4, 37, 40–2, 43, 45, 66, 80
self-help groups 122–3
self-isolating 121, 123
shaping the market 11, 33, 43, 68,
    69–72, 111
Shared Lives 107
shareholders 53, 95, 100
Sharpe, L.J. 85
short-term resource pressures 43
siloed working 32, 88
Simpson, P. 77–8
Skills for Care 55, 57, 59, 113–14
small and medium-sized
    enterprises 109
small-scale operators 104–5
Smith et al 10
'social bath' 139
social capital 49, 105
Social Care, Department of 98
Social Care Enterprise Agency 98
Social Care Futures 107, 142
Social Care Inspectorate 98
social care precept 76, 77
Social Care Sector COVID-19 Support
    Task Force 128
social care tax 82
Social Care Training Council 98
Social Care Wales 98
social contract approach 94–5, 96,
    100, 109

social enterprise sector 110–11
social impact 102
social insurance 81–2
social isolation 107
social justice 91
social networks 106
social rights 139
social security 17, 18
social services departments 9–10, 16,
    19, 49
Social Services Inspectorate 140
social value 101–2, 103
social value organisations 103, 104
social work 20, 29, 93
Social Work England 98–9, 126
social workers 9, 12, 13, 39
    and Barclay Report 20, 21
    registration 126
    training 57–8
Somerset 108
the South East 78
Southern Cross 50–1, 66, 68
the South West 108
Special Transitional Grant 18
spending
    buying goods and services from
        external suppliers 16
    local authority 4, 50
    reductions 54
stability, and well-being 109
staff buyouts 23
staffing 35, 96, 97–8, 103, 105, 120
    see also workforce
stakeholders 94, 96, 109, 137
the state, diminishing the role of 11–12
State of Caring Survey 44
status 55–8, 97–9, 113, 138
statutory duties, easement of 124–
    6, 129
statutory sector 20, 25, 28, 30
steering 28
Stewart, J. 83
stockholder theory 94, 96
strategic misrepresentation 137
strategic role, commissioning 35
The Structure of Scientific Revolutions
    (Kuhn) 144
Studdert, J. 114
Sunrise Senior Living 68
supplementary benefit 17
support grant, adult social care 76
Sutherland Report 82, 139

T

'task and time' model 60
taxation 11, 82–3
taxation-funded payments 28–9

tax havens 53
tendering 15, 31, 102–3
Thatcher government 11–12, 19, 29
third sector 25, 30, 36–7, 103, 121–4
  see also voluntary sector
Thomas, C. 131
Thompson et al 146
'time and task' approach 71
Timmins, N. 8, 10, 138
Titmuss, Richard 136–7
top-up payments 40, 79–80
Total Place 88
Towns Fund 85
Toynbee, P. 42
Trade Union Council 96
trade unions 56, 97, 99
traditional owner/managers 27, 30
training 55, 57–8, 99, 101
transformational co-production 106
transport volunteers, NHS 123
travelling time 54
Tronto, J. 92
Troubled Families 88
trust 43, 45
Tunstill, J. 58
turnover rates, staff 59, 60
Tussell 102

U

UK2070 Commission 84
unethical business behaviour 100
unethical policy and practice 117,
  128–31
Unison 99
United Nations Convention on
  the Rights of Persons with
  Disabilities 101
University of Birmingham 33
unmet need 43–4, 45, 79
unpaid carers 44, 79
Unwin, Julia 60, 93, 136
Unwin Inquiry 105
upfront information 67
US 135
user-led organisations (ULOs) 106

V

vacancies, social care 58
validation 142, 143
'values-based' approach 99

veil of ignorance 82
Victorian social policy 7, 8, 14
virtue ethics 91
voluntary sector 7, 23, 24, 27, 30,
  43–4, 49
  and commissioning 36–7, 45, 104
  and fragility 121–4
volunteers 49, 107, 123, 132
vulnerable people 50, 61, 66, 87–
  8, 107
  and Covid-19 120, 129, 130

W

wages 96–7
  see also pay
Wales 98, 99, 103–4
Walker, D. 42
wealth building, local 109
wealth tax 83
wealthy areas 49, 66
welfare, promotion of 91
welfare institutions 8
welfare state approach 20
well-being 91, 99, 100–4, 109
Wellbeing of Future Generations
  Act 103–4
Welsh Co-operative Centre 110
We Own It 64
White Paper 1989 19–20, 25
Why Local Democracy? (Sharpe) 85
The Wigan Deal 108
Williams, Bernard 94
winter fuel payments 82
Wistow, G. 17
Wistow et al 22–5, 31
Wootton, Barbara 12, 13
worker ownership models 109
workforce 1, 48, 53–61, 96–
  100, 120–1
  and Covid-19 118, 125, 131
  and security 65
working-age adults 1, 8

Y

younger adults 1, 3–4
Younghusband, Eileen 12

Z

zero-hours contracts 55, 56, 59, 97, 99,
  120–1